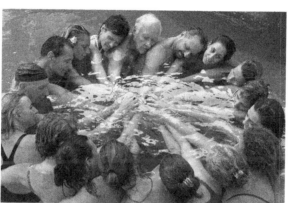
© IRENO GUERCI

Other books by Harold Dull
include:
    Tantsu a Yoga of the Heart (2008)
    Watsu® *Freeing the Body in Water* 4th Edition (2008)
    Finding Ways to Water *Collected Poems 1955-2007* (2007)
    Bodywork Tantra (1987)
    The Star Year (1967)
    The Door (1964)
    The Wood Climb Down Out Of (1962)
    Bird Poems (1958)

His DVDs
include:
    Watsu 1
    Watsu 2
    Watsu 3
    Tantsu® and Home Spa Watsu
    Tantsu Core Cradles
    Watsu Explorer Path and Tantsuyoga

Order from www.watsu.com

    Watsu® and Tantsu® are service marks registered in the name of Harold Dull

Copyright © 2018 by Harold Dull

All rights reserved, including the right to reproduce this book or portion thereof in any form without the written permission of the author.

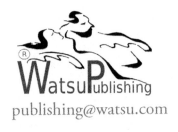

publishing@watsu.com

WATSU®
Basic and Explorer Paths

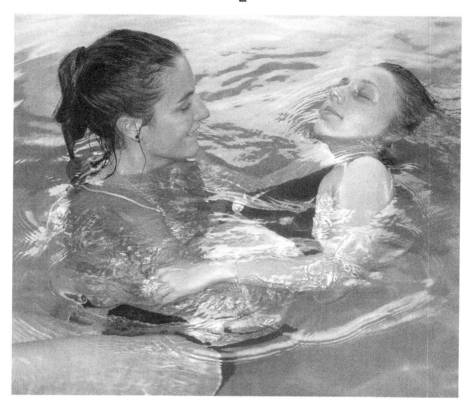

on Land and in Water
Harold Dull

with

Minakshi, Fabrizio Dalle Piane and Ateeka

The Creative Engagement of our Life Force

CONTENTS

About the Author	6
Acknowledgments	6
Preface	7

INTRODUCTION — 10
Preparations	11
The Float Test	13
The Watsu Pool	13

WATSU BASIC PATH — 14

Lesson 1 Waterbreath Dance — 15
Solo	15
Opening a Session	16
First Float	17
Closing a Session	18
Continuity	18

Lesson 2 Offerings — 19
Traction	19
Simple Offering	20
One Leg Offering	20
Two Leg Offering	21
The Diagonal Vector	21

Lesson 3 Accordions — 22
Opening and Closing	22
Rotate/Spiral Accordion	23
Free Spine	23

Lesson 4 Explore Flow — 24
Gate Hold	24
Explore Flow	25

Lesson 5 Return to the Breath — 27
Distant Stillness	27
Seaweed to the Other Side	28

TRANSITION FLOW — 29
Near Leg Rotation	30
Far Leg Rotation	30
Arm Breath Squeeze	30
Hand Hold	31
Pull Around	31
Swing	31
Push Around	32
Arm Leg Rock	32
Thigh Press	32
Turn and Pull	32
Sweep Under Shoulder	33
Lengthening Spine	33
Spine Pull	34
Undulating Spine	34
One Turn And Pull	34
Side Saddle	34
Sandwich	35
Head Lift	35
Sandwich 2	36
Explore Movement	36
Heart Rock	36

Precautions	37
New Watsu & Tantsu by Minakshi	39

POWER OF THREE — 42
Watsu Round	43

WATSU EXPLORER PATH
- The Themes and the Flow ... 50
- Format ... 51
- Explorer Tandem Watsu ... 52
- Origins ... 53
- Station 1 Basic Elements ... 54
- Station 2 Breath Shift ... 56
- Station 3 Saddles ... 58
- Station 4 Cradles ... 60
- Station 5 Overgrip ... 62
- Station 6 Presses ... 64
- Station 7 Accordions ... 66
- Station 8 Knee and Foot ... 68
- Station 9 Wall and Steps ... 70
- Station 10 Catches ... 72
- Station 11 Side Tandem ... 74
- Station 12 Whole Tandem ... 76

TANDEM WATSU ... 78
- Preparation ... 79
- Orchestration ... 79
- Watsu for two by three ... 83

TANTSUYOGA ... 89
- Water Flower ... 90
- Seven Celebrations ... 91
- Tandem Tantsuyoga ... 95
- Tantsuyoga Presenterships ... 97

TANTSU ... 98
- Posterior Cradle ... 99
- Anterior Cradle ... 100

ON THE PATH ... 104
- Other Paths that led to Watsu ... 105
- Learning from the Sequence ... 106
- Learning from the Flow ... 106
- The Path Back ... 107

FABRIZIO AND ATEEKA
- Art of the Somatic Dialogue ... 108
- Vital Importance of the Pause ... 110
- Participatory Witness ... 113
- Play, Humor and Pleasure ... 115
- The Regenerative Potential ... 119
- Neural Networks of Intelligence ... 121

HOME SPA WATSU ... 127

EXPLORATIONS
- Nurturing, Bonding, Intimacy ... 135
- Poetics of Watsu ... 138
- Boundlessness of Water ... 139
- Watsu and Continuum ... 140
- Pools I Have Stepped Into ... 140
- Stepping out of the Pool ... 141
- A Separate Path ... 142
- At the Heart of Watsu ... 144
- Woga ... 146
- Creative Movement ... 148
- Meridians Streaming ... 152
- Centers Resonating ... 154
- The Right Person ... 156
- On the Origens of Watsu ... 157

APPENDIX
- Worldwide Registry ... 163
- Books and DVDs ... 164
- WABA ... 166
- Afterwords ... 166

About the Author

Harold Dull was born in 1935 in Seattle and on graduation from the University of Washington in 1957, joined the poets who formed the San Francisco Renaissance where several of his books were published. After two years in Europe and three in Mexico City, in 1976 he began to study Zen Shiatsu, both in America and with its creator, Shizuto Masunaga, in Japan. In 1980 he began teaching Zen Shiatsu at a hot springs in Northern California and applied its stretches while floating his students in a warm pool. This evolved into the Watsu that is now used around the world in clinics and spas. For 35 years Harold has traveled to teach Watsu and Tantsu. He has taught in 30 countries, almost all the countries of Europe, and Brazil, Costa Rica, Mexico, Chile, Japan, Korea, Australia, New Zealand, India and Israel. He has studied several languages. He developed and maintains a Registry on the web that stores the transcripts of those from 95 countries who have studied Aquatic Bodywork and Tantsu and lists authorized practitioners, instructors and classes. He continues to be involved in the creation and production of his videos and books. When he is not traveling to teach he lives with his wife in Berkeley.

Acknowledgements

The first version of this book, and the new paths that have been developed for it, was a result of being asked in 2009 for a book on Watsu to accompany my Tantsu book that had just been published in Italy. Italo Bertolasi took most of its photographs, in an indoor pool in Milan, a pool by the ocean in Yelapa, Mexico and a pool in Auroville, India. Four pictures were taken in Auroville by Indio Guerci. Marcus Miller helped correct the images for publication. This current version started as the seventh edition of that first, but to better serve our students, we expanded this to include material of value from a textbook no longer in print.

Fabrizio Dalle Piane, who had helped develop the new core Tantsu, joined me in our first Watsu Tantsu Explore Flow classes in Italy and Mexico and helped develop the format of the Explorer Path. Ateeka joined us to insightfully explore the concepts our work calls up. The eagerness with which students in both classes welcomed this new path is appreciated, as well as the continuing support of all our water family in Italy, and that of students and instructors in other countries where I fine tuned its format.

As in all our endeavors, my wife and daughter provided support. For the six subsequent editions: Teachers and students around the world helped perfect the new Basic. Minakshi and Giordana Valli helped me come up with a new form of Tandem Watsu. Fabrizio Buffa, Italo and Simon Bolivar helped with its illustrations. Simon's video was a source for the TantsuYoga illustration. Instructors and students in Italy and wherever else we offered the Rounds helped develop them. The Watsu Round as something complete in itself was first introduced at Watsu Mexico. Mary Seamster and Cristina Levi provided wonderful pools and places for many of this book's illustrations in Washington state and Tuscany. . *HD*

PREFACE

Watsu is

- ### Therapy
Watsu alleviates a multitude of conditions, particularly those related to stress and/or isolation.

- ### Bodywork
Having our body treated as a whole activates our self healing.

- ### Paths of Personal Growth for both Holder and Held
All three appear to some degree in every Watsu. This book's Watsu Round adds a fourth:

- ### Community
Sharing and helping each other learn in threes strengthens our connections.

In 1980, at Harbin Hot Springs in Northern California, I floated someone in a warm pool and applied the stretches and principles of the Zen Shiatsu that I had studied with its creator in Japan. I had no idea that what was coming into being would help millions of children and others in clinics and spas around the world, and would become a new way to bring people together to come to know and celebrate their connection.

When I started applying Zen Shiatsu's principle of 'being not doing' unconditionally holding others, I was surprised by how much oneness I felt with each one floating at my heart, even those I would never have imagined being one with. Some said they too felt a oneness, that being held without intention had been missing from their lives. I saw Watsu as 'healing our wounds of separation'. Thousands of Watsus later, I am no longer surprised. Watsu frees us from the illusion of separation.

The being held that being floated necessitates accesses an older level of healing than that of touch. When infants fall a mother's response is to pick them up and hold them. Containment creates safety. Containment and safety reach new levels in this book's Rounds and Tandems.

We saw benefits come to both those floating, and to those being floated. Many practitioners and instructors speak of how Watsu changed their lives.

It changed mine. I realized that once we developed our program to train professionals, on what I call the vertical dimension, we need to bring its benefits to everybody on the horizontal dimension.

In thirty years the professional program is established. There are a hundred Watsu Instructors around the world. Students from 95 countries have transcripts on the Registry. Watsu instructors and practitioners have their own member association. Many are helping assemble a book, Watsu Professional Path, that details every Watsu move and its application and adaptation. It will accompany this book that presents Watsu's basic moves, and ways to bring Watsu's benefits to everybody sharing in threes on land and in water.

The year I started Watsu, I brought it's unconditional holding and containment back onto land in Tantsu. This book is a textbook for Basic Watsu, the Watsu Transition Flow, Tandem Watsu, Home Spa Watsu, and Core Tantsu. It has step by step instructions for teaching your friends while joining them in Tantsuyoga and Watsu Rounds. and for joining them on the Explorer Path, where three take turns exploring all the ways a theme or move can be done with the receiver giving constant feedback. Then all three take turns in a round in which each incorporates their theme.

The moves that I selected and adapted to open the round on the Explorer Path, turn out to be a major improvement over our previous Basic Watsu. After I got our team of Watsu Instructor's help in fine tuning and approving them, the new Basic Watsu took its place alongside the Explorer Path in the first edition of this book. The moves from two sides at the end of each turn in the round led to Tandem Watsu and the Watsu of Two by Three in this book's second edition which takes couple's work to a new level.

While teaching in India I was told that yoga means union. Realizing the new Tantsu was more a celebration of union than bodywork, I introduced it as Tantsuyoga.

In 2011, I was invited to present Tantsuyoga at the International Yoga Festival in Milan. Wishing to engage as many participants as possible, and having appreciated the power of rounds in our classes, I introduced a third role into Tantsuyoga. This third, a guide, positioned behind the holder to support his lower back, allowed the holder to keep his eyes closed and stay longer in the bottom of the breath. I introduced this Round to countless groups in Europe, America and South America. Everywhere people of all ages were profoundly moved by having their breathing engaged as they celebrate different levels of union with their eyes closed. This Flower Round, and the Water Flower that participants start it with, is featured in the third edition. In each subsequent edition I introduced new ways it could be combined and presented.

In the sixth edition I introduced the Ocean Within. In a class in which I encouraged students to bring the movement as water into Tantsuyoga, I suggested that the guide at my back also move as water. I realized that the three of us had joined in a state of being that can best be described as oceanic, a state in which each of us comes to know our Ocean Within, the whole that is greater than the sum of all the movements within.

This seventh edition, adds the Watsu Round, and how those who have learned it can lead their friends and family through it, taking turns as Holder, Helper and Held. The ease with which the Watsu Round can be shared, and the completeness of its experience, make it a big step towards realizing the potential that came into being in 1980. This version also adds Home Spa Watsu which brings benefits of Watsu to those who have no access to a pool. It adds observations and discoveries that accompanied the more than thirty years development of Watsu and Tantsu. A second volume, *Watsu Professional Path*, adds details about the applications and adaptations of Watsu and all its moves,

The additions to each edition open up new ways of looking at what went before without negating what accompanied the earlier creations. Those earlier ways remain as palimpsests, the even more ancient texts found under ancient writings. There is not a single path through this book. Explore it in any order. It does not matter if you read the palimpsest first or the text that was written over it. Each has its time as the only text and both continue to exist. The path that is before is the path that was behind. Two palimpsests that continue to exist under this book are the books, Watsu *Freeing the Body in Water* and Tantsu *a Yoga of the Heart*. Underlying them are whatever similar ideas have been expressed by others, and my own earliest writings, the poems that go as far back as twenty years before Watsu came into being. Poetry was my first Explorer Path. Unlike much of today's poetry which is a performance of what people want or ought to hear, poetry has been for me an exploration of what we don't know we know, as is this book.

PREFACE

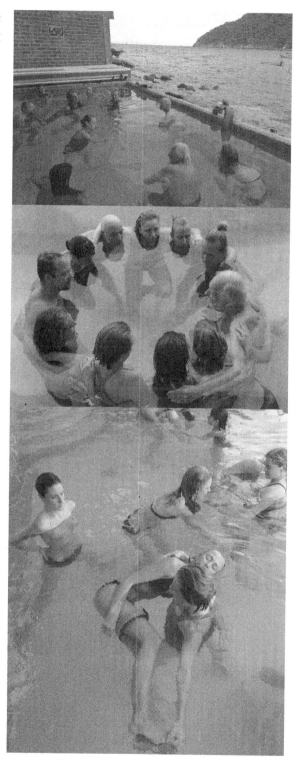

The first 36 pages of this book focus on the moves and principles taught in our beginning Watsu classes. Basic Watsu and Watsu Transition Flow (offered together as Watsu 1). Find a class at www.watsu.com. The only place where all authorized Watsu instructors list classes.

The power of three meets the power of water in the rest of this book which explores all the ways three can explore together and how the reader can introduce and share moves with a couple of freinds in rounds of three, both in water and on land.

Start on land with the Tantsuyoga (Watsu on land) on page 95 or in a pool with the Watsu Round on page 42. The Tantsuyoga can be shared anywhere; in the park, on the floor or at a massage table. The space you need in a warm pool for a round is less than that needed for an individual session. If a pool is not readily available, practicing Tantsuyoga, besides being complete in itself, prepares you for any subsequent sharing in a pool.

This book provides directions and scripts with which you can lead the others while you are within a round of three. Those who learn this well with you, can, with the help of this book, lead two others through a Round, helping fulfill our goal of making the benefits of both receiving and giving Watsu and/or Tantsu accessible to everybody, something very much needed in today's world.

Once you've learned Watsu's basic moves, you can join others on this book's Explorer Path. If two of you learn to work together well, you can start treating your freinds to this book's Tandem Tantsuyoga or Tandem Watsu.

CELEBRATE UNION

Help us get the benefits that come with all of the roles in our Rounds out to everybody.

WATSU

Watsu grew out of Zen Shiatsu. Shiatsu, like Acupuncture, balances the flow of energy in our bodies. Shizuto Masunaga, who created Zen Shiatsu, says that stretching is the oldest way to balance that flow. I studied with Masunaga in Japan and started teaching

Zen Shiatsu at Harbin Hot Springs in Northern California. In 1980 I explored applying the stretches and principles of Zen Shiatsu while floating my students in warm water. In the years since, with the help of countless others in classes, clinics and spas around the world, Watsu has evolved into what many consider the most profound development in bodywork in our time. While other modalities are based on touch, the holding that working in water necessitates, brings both the giver and the receiver to new levels of connection and trust. This, combined with the therapeutic benefits of warm water, the greater freedom of movement it encourages and the way it facilitates our application of Zen Shiatsu's most basic principle, that of being not doing, creates a modality that can affect every level of our being.

In thirty years Watsu has spread to every corner of the world. It has become a primary modality in Aquatic Therapy. Those we have authorized to teach Watsu have added to our Worldwide Registry students from more than ninety-five countries (I have taught in thirty).

The fifty-hour courses on Watsu's professional path, include Watsu 1 which combines Basic Watsu and the Transition Flow to smoothly bring someone into and out of Watsu's cradles, positions in which we brace someone's body with our own to stretch and work with them. In Watsu 2 students learn to adapt and expand the form with additional bodywork in each cradle. In Watsu 3 students learn to go beyond the form with advanced cradles and rolls that can lead into Free Flow. Advanced classes focus on clinical applications. In Watsu 4 practitioners go deeper into Free Flow and Tandem Watsu. Instructors teach students to adapt to a wide range of body types and situations. For more information, go to www.watsu.com where all the authorized instructors and classes are posted.

The Basic Path

A simple progression of moves and how to support and keep both your own body and that of whomever you float comfortable and aligned can be learned in our two-day Basic Watsu workshops offered around the world.

Until you are actually in the water with someone floating in your arms, or have been floated, it is hard to imagine. The first thing someone being floated notices is the closeness and the safety being held instills. The floater notices the unique kind of support the water provides and realizes what it means to let the water do everything, to just be with someone.

Wait in the emptiness at the bottom of each breath until the getting lighter of the one in your arms draws your breath up, draws you up out of that emptiness. The connection this establishes moves on to where everything moves to the breath as you continually traction a spine freed from the pressure gravity places upon it.

When those first opening moves bring you to a stillness, you may become aware of how close to your heart the one in your arms floats. With some, movements arise spontaneously through your heart and out your arms. With others. you wait and explore, moving as water. However the movements start, they enter a continuum as you change the position of your arms in a slow dance that engages your whole body and the ocean within and brings you to an even deeper stillness. The more family and friends you share this simple but complete progression of moves with, the more you will realize the oneness you feel with whoever is in your arms is your oneness with everything, is the path.

Energy

Before I brought the stretches of Zen Shiatsu into the water, I had learned to feel the energy being released by those stretches on land. In the water, where the stretches can be even more powerful, I began to move people around to the flow of what I felt those stretches release. This evolved into Free Flow. There are moments in Free Flow when we are moved into and out of positions without any idea of why or how.

Since every level of our being can become engaged in a Watsu, there is no way to identify or chart all the kinds of energy that we find flowing through and around us in a Watsu. It is there to discover. Just as the unconditional love that doesn't come into being when someone tells us to feel it, is there to discover when we feel our oneness with someone.

While developing the new Basic Watsu I got help fine-tuning it from countless Watsu instructors around the world, who voted that it should replace the old Basic Watsu.

The new opening was not moves selected from parts of a longer sequence like the old Basic Watsu. It remains the sequence of moves that open every Watsu. Students learn to be with the one in their arms well enough to go out and share it with family and friends. Each sharing takes them deeper into Watsu's potential. Its breath-timed moves are followed by the movement-as-water, the continuum that had previously not appeared until Watsu 3.

Precautions and Preparations

The precautions below should be observed by everybody. Listed among them are preparations useful for sharing Basic Watsu with someone who has never had a Watsu.

You should not watsu people who have a condition that precludes being in warm water for a period of time. Before a session, familiarize yourself thoroughly with the person and any conditions which might be worsened by pressure or movement. If there are any neck or back problems, find out if there are any movements that might have activated it in the past and avoid those movements. Avoid pressure or excessive movement of any area where inflammation is involved such as a sprain or tendonitis. More precautions are listed on page 38.

Always make it clear that people should inform you during a session of any discomfort and that you are willing to stop a session anytime they want. We must take the same care supporting our partner's head as we would the head of a newborn infant. As the muscles in the neck become more relaxed, the danger of hyperextension, of over compressing the disks and nerves between the vertebrae when the head falls back is increased. At the beginning one arm supports under the head just above the occipital ridge, maintaining a slight traction, while the other supports under the point between the sacrum and the top of the legs where their weight balances. Using flotation cuffs if the legs tend to sink, helps protect the neck, as well as the back. Stay aware of how you support the head throughout the session.

Keep the nose out of the water. If it does go under, as sometimes happens, keep calm. Bring the head to a vertical position so the water can drain out. Some people ride lower in the water than others. You can't watsu someone with their ears out of the water. Most people who are apprehensive relax and enjoy the feeling and the silence. Many are bothered by water sloshing in and out of their ears. Have ear plugs available. When first putting someone's ears under leave them submerged for three or four minutes. Rinsing the ears after a session with a combination of alcohol and white vinegar helps prevent swimmer's ear.

Some people may force a slow breathing. Others who have had experience with Rebirthing may keep up a rapid breathing which can lead to tetany, a spasmodic tightening of the muscles due to hyperventilation. In either case the person can be told to breathe normal deep breaths. If tetany spontaneously occurs, you may need to assure someone unfamiliar with this state, that it, and the tingling sensation that accompanies it, will go away by itself.

Except in circumstances like the above, or in cases of inappropriate behavior, it is better not to interrupt the process verbally. If you notice tears forming in someone's eyes, or sighing, or some other emotional reaction, continue the session. Give whatever is coming up the opportunity to work itself out in the flow of the Watsu. Watsu affects every level of our being. The intimacy of its holds can bring unanticipated issues to the surface. To truly be with someone be clear of any intentions. If they choose to remain silent after a session do not pressure them to share. For many Watsu provides a safe space in which emotions that have not been fully dealt with can arise and be let go of by the heart mind. This may be happening behind the tears we sometimes see in a receiver's eyes. It may continue to happen when they have been returned to the wall. Any questioning as to what happened or is happening may interrupt a deep healing process. But if the receiver feels the need to discuss something coming up, be a supportive listener and, if an issue warrants it, encourage the receiver to seek professional help.

Some people sink more than others. Muscle tends to sink and fat float. Hence women, who have more subcutaneous fat than men, tend to be better floaters. The more muscular someone is the more likely you will need to use flotation cuffs and adapt your positions. The closer you bring someone's center of gravity to your own line of gravity, and the less spread out their weight, the easier they are to support.

When I started Watsu flotation devices were not around. We gravitated to steps and positions such as cradles and saddles in which our body provided support. The development of float cuffs was welcomed. When needed, wrap them just above the knees. Avoid over-floating, which is indicated by the knees bobbing out of the surface. This makes it difficult to connect to the breath.

Float cuffs can be ordered through www.watsu.com.

INTRODUCTION

The Float Test

Many who receive their first Watsu have difficulty letting go when they lie back in the water. Some come out of a session in which their legs never bent once saying it was the most relaxed they have ever been. It does make our work easier when they let their legs go. And it increases the benefits they receive. You can introduce the following float test before you start someone's first Watsu session.

Tell someone you want to see what size floats they might need and attach float cuffs just above the knees, a size that brings their knees just to the surface, level with their pelvis.

Then say: *People float differently depending on what state they are in. I want to see how you float in two different states. When you first lie back over my arm I want you to close your eyes, press your arms to your side and extend and lengthen your legs. Hold that for at least three breaths. Then I want you to go as limp as you can. Notice where my arms support you. Feel free now, or anytime during the Watsu, to move them to where it would be more comfortable.*

Float them and when you stand them up, ask how comfortable they had felt. Check if they had any discomfort. If so discuss the probable causes and adjust your session accordingly.

Express appreciation for any adjustment they made (which your arm stores for future use). Tell them they can make adjustments anytime it would increase their comfort during the session and that they are free to move their body if needed, to lift their head if it begins to feel strain laying back, etc.

Ask how it felt being in the two states. Point out that the more they stay in the second state, the more they will get out of their session. (If you feel it might be needed later you can introduce a cue you might use to get them to bend a leg, such as lifting up under the knee, etc.)

The Watsu Pool

The ideal Watsu pool has many levels so that the practitioner can work with a person at a variety of depths. In a single session pool with one depth, the ideal is two-thirds the practitioner's height. In deeper pools practitioners become limited in how wide they can spread their legs, and how deep they can sink into the breath. In shallower pools moves that bring someone to a vertical position become difficult, but in a somewhat shallow pool you may find it easier to support someone with your legs or knees.

The larger (and less crowded) the pool the better. You need space to turn someone without their feet touching the wall, a circle at least twelve feet in diameter.

The water temperature should be about the same as the body's surface temperature (94° Fahrenheit, 35° centigrade), one or two degrees warmer if the temperature of the air over the pool is colder. Drink copious amounts of water to avoid dehydration.

There should be no background music. Its rhythms block connecting to the breath and mask our inner rhythms.

If you don't have a pool to work in, explore what is available locally for training babies to swim or for treating people with special needs. Many students find volunteering their services at such places to be particularly rewarding.

Many Watsu Practitioners have their own individual session pool that they are willing to rent to others. One advantage to meetings on the explorer path is that a pool large enough for a single session can serve for a meeting of three (six in the Watsu Round). Once you've taken a class, you will have access to the pools that others list on our Registry.

For information about pool construction and maintenance: **watsu.com/watsu_pools.pdf**

WATSU BASIC PATH

Many entry-level Watsu instructors first introduce Watsu's basic moves in the Watsu Round. They have students practice the kind of movement, grounding and alignment that will aid their watsuing and being with others. Many introduce Tantsuyoga which brings Watsu's unconditional holding and engagement with the breath onto land. Both Rounds take you deeper the more you practice them.

Instructors check each student's head support and alignment of the one in their arms. They also encourage those being floated to give feedback and help the floater perfect his support. Having this instruction and feedback from the beginning, lessens the likelihood of developing habits that would be later hard to correct and could cause discomfort or injury.

Being in a class with other students provides a range of body types to learn with and leads to having others to practice with after the class, both your classmates and those that list their availability on the Registry which, once you take a class, you have access to. You also have access to listed pools and can list your own availability for exchanges.

Core Engagement

On land in dance, martial arts and other body oriented modalities our core has its center in the abdomen where we ground and move from, our Body Center. In water, where the water supports us as much as the ground under our feet, when we float someone on the surface at our heart, a second core center comes into play, our Heart Center. Besides being a progression of the moves in Basic Watsu, in these opening moves there is the changing engagement within of our core's two centers.

Every Watsu begins with dropping into the emptiness at the bottom of the breath and staying there, doing nothing, until the one on our arms gets lighter as they breathe in. Their getting lighter draws our breath up, draws us up out of the emptiness. Repeatedly being drawn up establishes the rhythm that our own breath, that our own moves continue to move to, moves that cannot be stopped to check if they are still breathing to that rhythm.

In the opening these breath-timed moves build up to a point where we move beyond the breath and, clasping the hips, stop in stillness.

Stillness and Explore Flow

Stillness is not emptiness. Stillness is what whoever is at our heart floats on. It is the quietest form of love. As we stay in Stillness, doing nothing, not even sinking to the breath, we may sense some movement inside the one we float that we recognize as a call, an invitation for our movement to join. Or we may sense a movement or wave coming up through our heart and out our arms drawing us to move as water. Or we may feel drawn to explore different ways we can move with them;

Lesson 1 Waterbreath Dance

The Waterbreath Dance, surrendering to the water and being lifted by it without doing anything, opens every Watsu and establishes the breathing pattern underlying subsequent moves. It is done as a solo, as a duet when you face the one you are about to float in the opening of a session, and as the first move when you have someone in your arms. Included in this lesson is the way you will close every session with someone.

Solo

The more fluid we become in our own bodies, the more we can let the water do everything. Whenever you first step into a pool, settle into the water and surrender to whatever movement being in water draws you into.

Each of these lessons suggests ways that a solo dance can prepare you for the lesson's moves and principles. With this lesson explore how the water supports you, a support that will stay with you while you float someone.

Find a depth where, when you stand, the water is a little higher than your navel. Explore the contrast between our most non-fluid state and our most fluid. Stand up out of the water, your body stiffened. Then shake all that tension out of your body and settle down, your legs spread, your chin in the water. Feel the water become a chair supporting you.

Explore further the water's support by contrasting its complete support with a partial support. Stand close enough to a wall of the pool that you can reach out and lean lightly against the wall. Notice where there is a fulcrum where your weight and its support is centered between your feet on the bottom and your hand against the wall. Remove your hand from the wall and

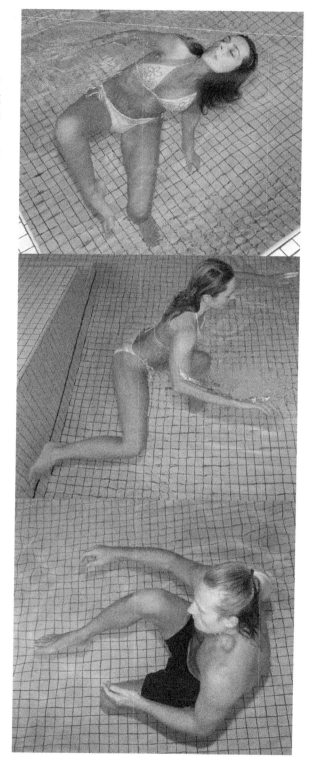

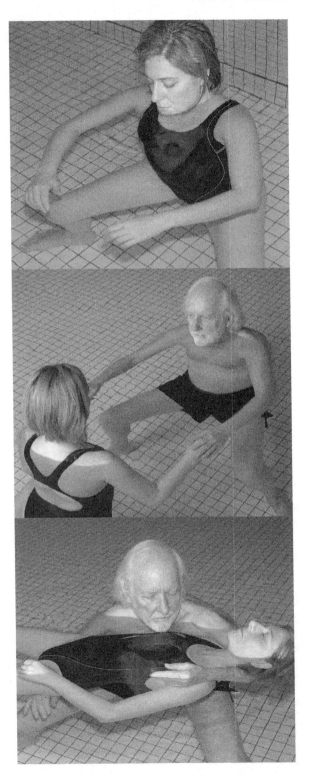

settle back into the water. Notice how peripheral the support becomes, your body supported from all sides by the water. Explore how that support helps balance you when you lift one foot up

Return to your settled stillness in the water, legs spread and relaxed, water up to your chin. Notice how as you breathe in, the water slowly lifts you towards the surface without you having to do anything and then the water settles you back down as you breathe out. Continue through several breaths dropping a little deeper into the emptiness at the bottom of each breath. This is called the Waterbreath Dance whether it is done alone or with someone floating in your arms.

Duet - Opening a session

If flotation cuffs are needed to keep the receiver's legs from sinking, fasten them just above the knees, the size that keeps their knees from bobbing out.

Ask the receiver to lean back against the wall in the most comfortable position possible with their feet spread. Tell them to focus on the straightness in their back and that, when they feel the support of the wall at their back again, they will know they're coming to the end of the session and they should focus again on that straightness.

Request them to step out and feel another kind of support, the support of the water. Facing them, tell them to do the same thing you do. Settle down in the water to your chin. Let the water lift you up with each breath. Tell them to surrender to the water. Don't hold their hands. You want them to surrender to the water, not you. Have your hands, palms down, floating over theirs ready to catch them if they start losing their balance. Tell them to close their eyes and let the water breathe them up. When they've let the water lift them a few times, and your breathing is coordinated, step to their right side and float them up into first position.

First Float

The first position is characterized by floating someone close, their right arm behind your back, your left arm reaching over it to support the head. Lift them into Position 1 with the back of your right hand under their right thigh, palm down. As the back of their head just above the occipital ridge comes to rest on the side of your bent elbow, slip your right forearm up to where you feel their weight balances on it. Someone's balance point could be at the top of their legs or under their buttocks or their tailbone. Let your left hand or its fingertips come to rest on their shoulder to keep their head aligned. Maintain a gentle traction and avoid contact with their neck. With a wide stance settle down in the water.

While floating someone notice how complete their letting go is. If the legs are stiffened, lift up under the knees to encourage them to unlock and return your arm to the balance point. Settle down into the emptiness at the bottom of the breath. Wait. When you feel the receiver's weight lessening on the arm that is under their balance point, breathe in as the water lifts both of you towards the surface. Avoid any rocking. Let their head rise with their body just enough to keep both ears in the water and avoid sloshing. Don't wait for them to breathe out and sink. Whenever ready, breathe out and wait at the bottom of the breath, the place where it is easiest to wait. Because most people breathe in faster than they breathe out, the bottom of the breath is where you can best perceive the change of weight on your arm. The more you practice this, the more you will feel the breath coming in draws you up out of a deeper and deeper emptiness, a non-doing so deep that even the doing of waiting disappears.

With those who don't sink, you can rest your forearm across their hara (abdomen) where your arm being lifted will draw your breath in.

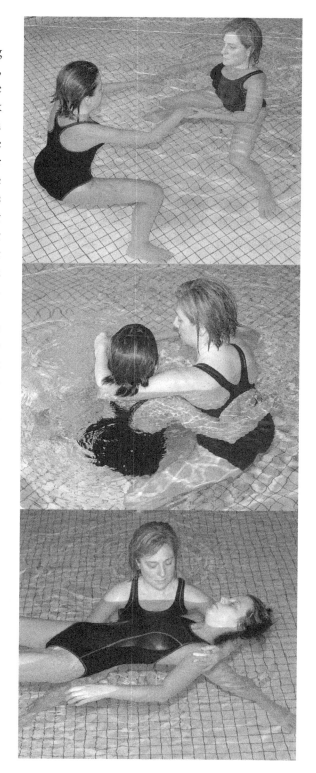

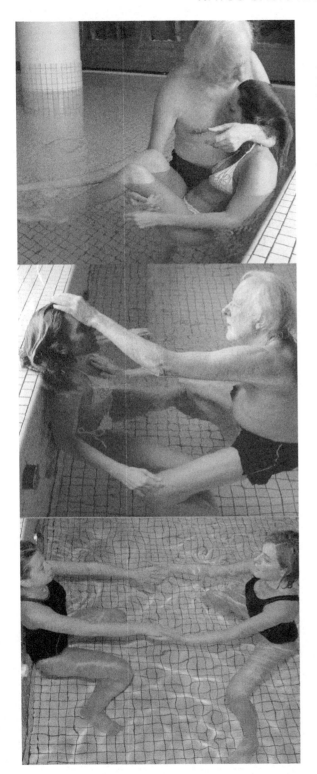

Closing a Session

Do the Waterbreath Dance close to the wall. Lift their head up with one forearm as the other lifts their knees, their back vertical. Rotate on the axis of your spine. Push the far leg down and away, and the near leg down towards you to give them a wide base as you lean their back against the wall. Gently place your right hand on their heart center. Your left hand gently holds their neck to release any tension and comes to rest very lightly on the third eye. Hold. Focus on whatever rising you feel up your own spine as you simultaneously lift both hands up. Lower your hands under theirs where your middle fingers lift their hands just to the surface. Move back and focus on how you are still connected though no longer touching. Be there when they open their eyes

Continuity

An essential element of Watsu is continuity, the seamless flow from move to move. Once the Waterbreath Dance has established the rhythm we will breathe and coordinate our subsequent movement to, once we start moving to that rhythm, we do not stop to make sure the receiver still breathes to it. That would break the flow, and if they have been unconsciously coordinating their breath to our movement, when we stop they may stop breathing and wait for us to move again. We do stop, but only when we feel whatever movement we have been doing has completed. At that moment when those in our arms also feel that completion they can drop deepest into the stillness out of which inner movement arises.

Enhance the continuity throughout the breath-coordinated opening moves by swiveling your feet over the same places while those in your arms imagine themselves being moved around the pool without the jolt of footsteps.

Lesson 2 Offerings

Traction

The Water Breath Dance establishes the rhythm of our breathing that we continue to move to. Another essential element of Watsu is the gentle spinal traction that, with practice, becomes automatically ingrained in the way we hold someone as we pull them through the water. This protects the neck and lower back from hyperextending. The more relaxed someone becomes lying on their back in warm water, the more their head should be supported as carefully as the head of a newborn.

Besides its value in protecting, there can be many positive benefits in traction. The buoyancy of water counters the effects of gravity on our spine. The pressure on nerves that have been compressed between the vertebrae can be relieved with traction. Other channels that service the whole body can become more open.

Traction is maintained through all the breath-timed moves of the opening.

Solo

Stand low in the water facing forward, your legs spread as wide as is comfortable. Keep your feet in the same place and your arms held out in front of you. Starting from your head, explore engaging more and more of your body as you turn slowly from side to side. Turn just the head. Then the shoulders, waist, knees, and feet. When you turn from the hips be sure your hara faces the side you turn toward. When your feet are engaged, your heels should be lifted as you slowly swivel on the balls of your feet.

Then coordinate the slow turning of your whole body to your breath. Do the solo WBD. Bending your right knee, settle down to that side as you breathe out. Push your right foot against

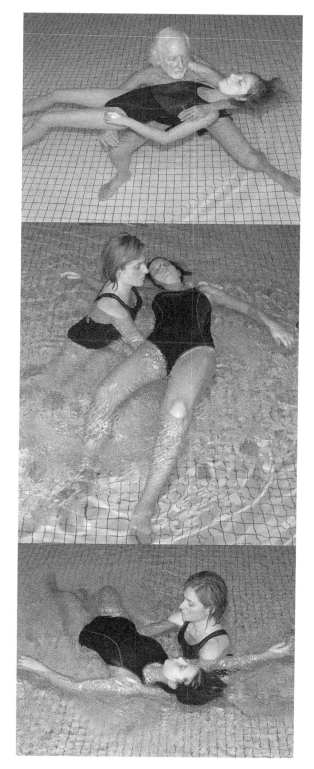

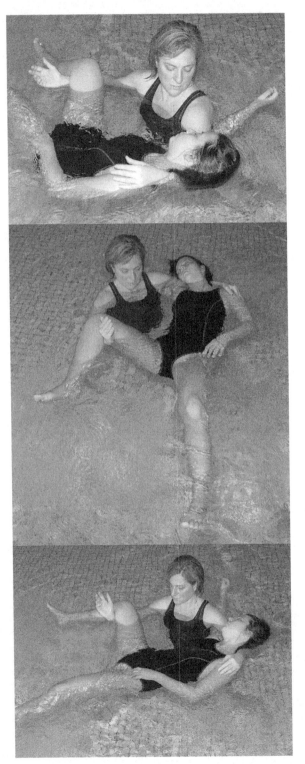

the bottom as you start to breathe in, causing your body to turn towards your left. Have your bent left arm up, a leading arm that the vector of force from your pushing foot arrives in. Whenever ready, breathe out as that arm keeps leading you around, and settle back on your right foot. As you breathe in push with the other foot to turn you back in the same manner to the side you started from, the vector from the foot you push arriving in the opposite arm, the one you lead with. Continue from side to side.

Simple Offering

Once you feel fully established in rising and settling with the breath in the WBD, the next time you start to settle, bend your right knee letting them slowly sink toward what we call our foot foot because it is on the same side as their feet. Each time you feel them start to get lighter, breathe in letting the breath bring you back up to center without any rocking over to the other side. Notice how there is a strength potential in your bent leg. The third time you breathe in push against the bottom initiating a vector of force that arrives in your opposite arm to traction your partner's occiput to the other side. Settle down to your head foot and, just before they come to a complete stop, push against the bottom and pull them back over your foot foot with the back of your hand hooking their far hip (or sacrum if it doesn't reach the hip). Their ears can come out of the water.

One Leg Offering

After pulling their body in a continuous loop from side to side at least three times, the next time you pull the head, leave your right arm behind until their knee floats over it. For the next three loops pull them by that leg folded across your arm. To continually maintain traction never push the leg as you pull the head.

Two Leg Offering

As you pull the head around with one arm, your arm that is still under their near leg scoops up the far leg. Pull the person by both legs each time you loop them away from the head.

As you continue from side to side coordinate all the offerings to your breath. As you pull to one side do not push with the other arm but maintain a constant traction. As you pull to a side don't wait until you get there to breathe out. Start breathing out whenever you feel ready to. As you are breathing out while the one in you arms continues floating around, settle down in a way that prepares you for the push with the other foot. Come from the foot foot to a still point facing center.

The Diagonal Vector

In all the breath-coordinated opening moves the feet stay over the same place, only their heels lifting as they change direction in the offerings. In the WBD we did not initiate any move but surrendered to the water lifting us together as the breath came in. This establishes the rhythm with which our breath will accompany subsequent moves. We do not interrupt that movement to wait for the other's breath. In all the offerings we explore how one move, our foot's push against the bottom can initiate movement that the breath continues to accompany. In all the offerings our body's engagement under the water is the same. When we are ready to breathe out, the one in our arms continues their float around as we settle down, preparing to push against the bottom with our other foot as we breathe in, setting up a vector of force that, arriving in our opposite arm, tractions the one we float. In the Solo we practice these movements to prepare for having someone in our arms.

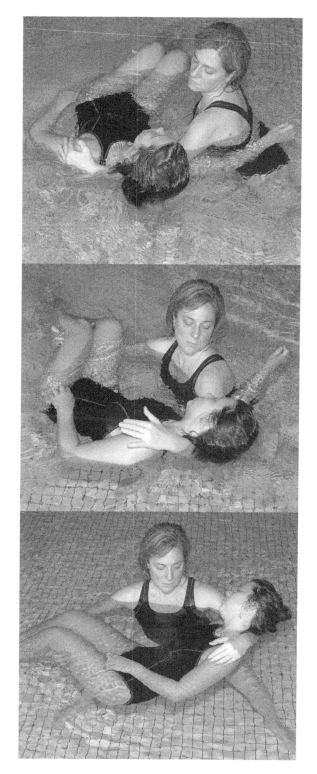

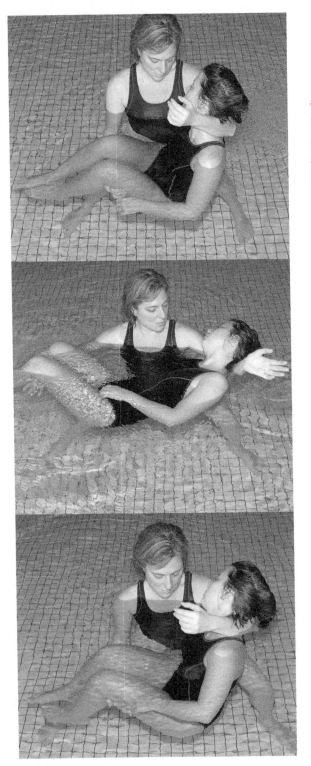

Lesson 3 Accordions

Solo

Stand facing forward, legs spread as wide as is comfortable. Do the solo WBD. Sink three times to the foot foot. Follow with the movements of the offerings from side to side. Stand with arms spread. As you breathe in open arms. As you breathe out lift up your left arm and bring your right towards the center beneath it. Continue. Face half way (45 degrees) towards your left foot. Keep your left arm steady in front of you as you move your right arm in a counter clockwise circle that approaches your left arm at each outbreath. At that approach rock your pelvis backward. Rock it forward as your circling arm approaches your chest. Simultaneously build up the speed of the circling and your breath. Hold your right arm out, palm down and push it out and back out and back faster than the breath.

Opening and Closing

In the Waterbreath Dance it was the void we kept dropping into until the other's breath drew us up. In the offerings that moment is shorter, a turning point in which a push against the bottom starts us back to the other side. In the accordion it is a hold, a press, until the breath comes in to open our arms.

Begin facing center in the position that the Two Leg Offering ends with, both knees comfortably over your right arm, a still point in which you wait to feel their breath coming in. When it does, open your arms wider and, as you breathe out, sink their hips to bring their legs closer to their chest. Continue opening the legs wider with each inbreath and bringing them closer to their chest with each outbreath, tractioning with a gentle pull of the head in both phases, upwards as you bring the legs towards the chest on the outbreath letting the hips sink, and outwards as you open the legs on the inbreath. Be sure there is no tight clasping of the neck in either phase.

Rotating/Spiraling Accordion

The movement in each stage brings us into new relationships to the breathing, the sinking and rising in the WBD, the turn and pull in the Offerings, the closing and opening in the Accordion. The relationship becomes more complex when we rotate the accordion, and still more complex when we are able to introduce a swing that, building up our breath's speed, becomes a spiraling that, suddenly released out straight, carries us beyond the breath.

As you press the knee to the chest in the accordion's last closing, place your left hand behind their left shoulder with your elbow still supporting their head and face 45 degrees towards your head foot (the foot nearest their head). Inscribe a counter clockwise circle with their knees pressing them towards their chest as you breath out. As you breathe in pull them towards you. If their hips tend to swing out, encourage that swing. Then rock your pelvis back to create a space for their hips to swing towards you. As you breathe out circle the knees back up. Let the swing, and the accompanying breath, gradually build up into a Spiraling Accordion.

If their size or condition makes swinging difficult, continue a Rotating Accordion turning towards the foot foot each time you open your arms.

Free Spine

(Spiraling +) When the spiraling to the breath reaches its maximum speed, the next time your arms open, facing center, straighten the spiraling out into strokes faster than the breath with your forearm under the sacrum.

(Rotating +) As you complete a final rotation open your arms. Slip your arm under the sacrum. Engaging your hips, move to your breath.

Stop suddenly and clasp the body gates.

In Free Spine the back of the arm, hand downwards, is never lifting the body up. Whenever movement within appears we follow it.

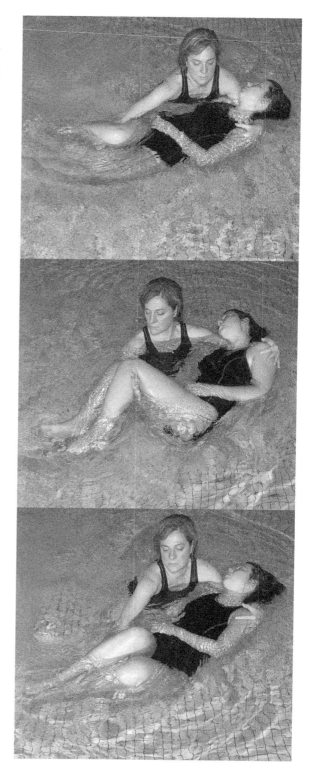

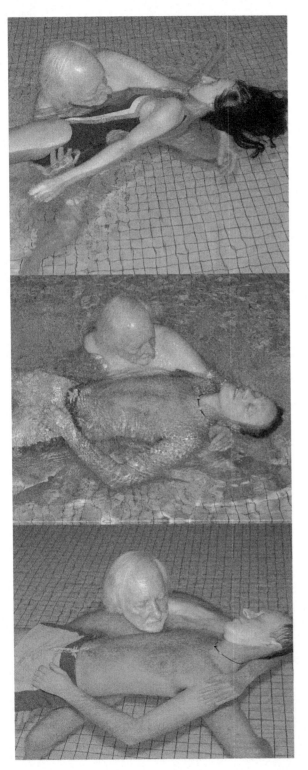

Lesson 4 Explore Flow

All the movements from the first when the breath that draws us up together out of the emptiness to Free Spine are connected to the breath. Breath-timed moves originate in the same center as do our moves on land. In water, as on land, our legs, and their connection to the earth, our grounding on the vertical dimension, support our breath-timed moves. In water, floating someone at our heart center, it becomes the center of moves on another dimension, moves that are not breath timed, but a continuum.

Solo

Stand up to your chin in the water, eyes closed. Notice how every part of your body responds to the movement in any part. If your arm floats out to one side, the opposite hip may dip to the other side to balance it. Be as water. Become water flowing out to all sides. Let your right hand, held half way out, fingers down, become a fixed point that, like a rock in a stream, all the water flows around. Reach out and around, your hand facing you. Become the water that surrounds, that contains.

Gate Hold

When the spine feels the freest in the Free spine, suddenly clasp their body gates between your right shoulder and the heel of your hand. These hollows of soft tissue next to the greater trochanters, are considered in India (along with those in the upper corners of the chest) to be gates where the spirit enters. Clasp as firmly as possible. Do not lift their body. If you can't lower your shoulder to the body gate, clasp it with your biceps. If your arm is not long enough to support the head, clasp with your right shoulder just high enough up from the gate to be able to support their head at the back of your wrist, fingers pointing up, palm facing out.

Maintaining the firm clasp of the gate, floating someone at your heart center, notice whatever tends to move out the arm under their head. The flow of the meridians in the arms is related to the heart. Our hearts resonate to those of others. Just as our legs ground us, our arms connect us to others. Feel yourself drawn out your arm. If not, focus on what is building up behind the Gate Hold. Release the hold and be drawn out into the movement as water, engaging your whole body in its continuum.

Explore Flow

When you are drawn out into movement through your arm that is under the head in the Gate hold, your other hand releases its hold and, palm down, moves in its own way. In moving as water, nothing is mirrored, nothing is repeated. Each arm goes its own way. Allowing every part of your body to join in its own way, to intertwine in this continuum, opens the Ocean Within, the whole that is greater than the sum of all the movements within. Be as water flowing out to all sides, rising up one moment and settling down and around the next. Explore a flow that has no end. Engage your whole body in whatever movement you begin exploring, slowly sinking to one leg or the other, or rising up out of the pool. Allow any movement you make to balance yourself and feed into the continuing exploration/flow. Do not be concerned about whether you have really entered into a flow or your movements are exploratory. In any case don't race out of the slow spacious movement that the heart feels most engaged in.

Heart Gate Flow

Without interrupting the flow, place the base of your left thumb in, or close to the opposite Heart Gate. The flow of the river within the one you hold joins the flow of the river within you.

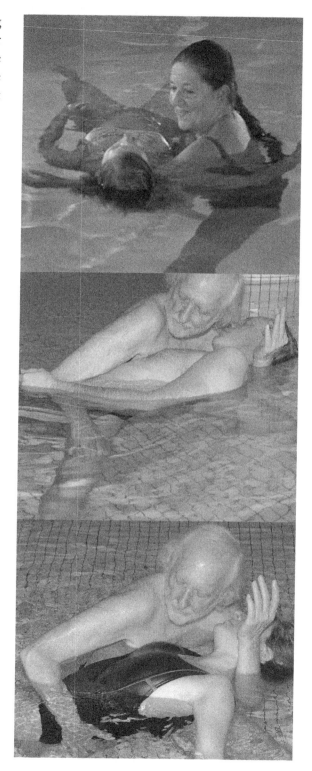

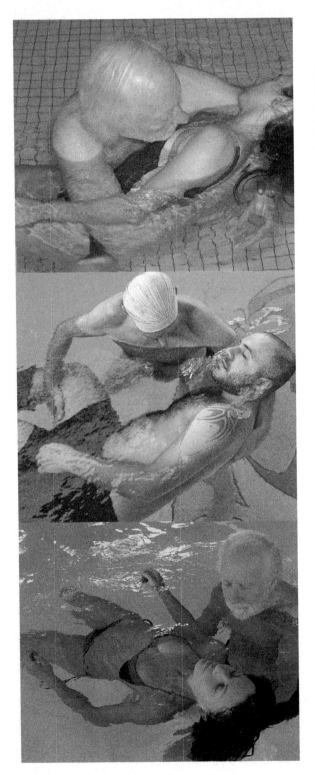

Near Gate Flow

Without interrupting the flow, with your arm bent place the heel of your right hand, fingers down, in the near Body Gate. Continue the movement as water, water that flows around the fixed point your hand in the body gate maintains. Do not push them away, but if they start to flow away, your hand in the heart gate can pull them over the fixed point.

Far Gate Flow

Without halting the flow, in one motion remove your hand from their body gate and reach up over their hara, hooking the opposite body gate, or as near as possible, with the heel or palm of your right hand. Notice how the reaching over brings them closer and more of your body becomes engaged. Explore how the side of your body and thigh can support and add to the containment, as well as the hand in the heart gate. Move as water that contains, contains you and all that you hold, the Ocean Within. Be moved together in that wholeness

Free Arm

Overgrip the thigh nearest you close to the knee and press it towards his chest while his head moves into your other hand and his arm slips out between you. If it doesn't, reach down and pull it out from behind your back up between you into the free float position, the head in one hand and their balance point in the other, palm up.

The more we practice on these paths, the more the flow enters into our lives outside the pool. The only techniques we bring onto this path are those that continue to open doors and windows to the flow.

Lesson 5 Return to the Breath
Solo

Move through the whole Progression up to this point. Become invisible. Feel how different it is to imagine someone out in your hands instead of on your arms close to your heart. Turn your palms to face each other and, keeping your arms straight, repeatedly turn your body to one side with the inbreath and to the other with the outbreath.

Distant Stillness

With both arms out straight let their head rest on one hand, open, palm up, while their body rests on the other, palm up under the balance point. Stay still. Do not try to connect to their breathing. Do not explore any movement or any connection from your heart. Do nothing. Disappear. The more invisible your hands are at the two ends of their spine, the more likely they are to get in touch with whatever moves up their spine. If you feel that movement between your hands, do nothing. The movement through their spine is whole in itself. Often an unwinding starts spiraling between our hands that is an honor to hold as a witness to the life in the core of another.

Seaweed

When the stillness seems complete, float the head across in front of your face and place it securely on your right shoulder. Holding their body gates with both hands move them slowly to the breath, their legs out in front swinging like seaweed from side to side. Be sure their head remains comfortably placed on your shoulder in a way that provides some traction. Do not continue in this position if their legs sink as it could hyperextend both their lower back and their neck. If your arms are not long enough to reach both body gates, press against one with one hand and the rib cage with the other.

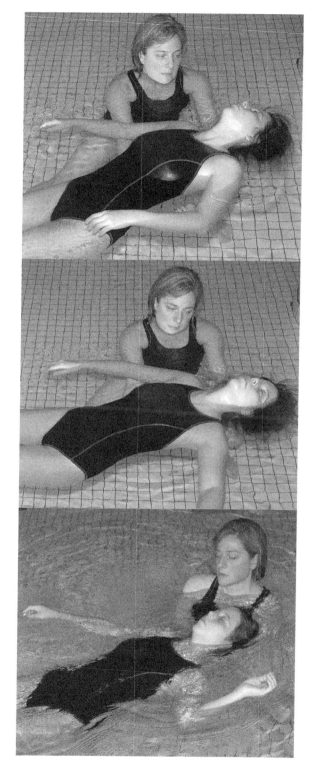

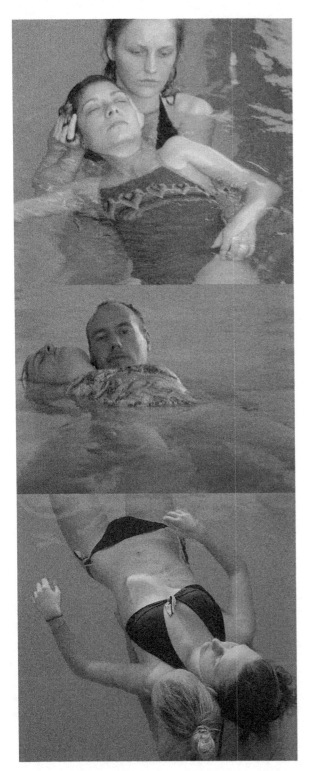

Going to the Other Side

To come out on their second side gradually lower your shoulder, floating their head into the crook of your right elbow that pulls them as you overgrip their near leg and maneuver them, adjusting your own position, until their left arm slips behind your back in first position. Alternatively, gently press your right hand against their upper back, turning them to face you, until their arm drops behind your back. Assist with your other hand if needed.

Starting from this new side go through the opening moves. When you get to the Distant Stillness use the seaweed to return to the first position on their right side and do the Waterbreath Dance. You can close at the wall or you can start a new cycle. It usually takes about twenty minutes to do both sides of a cycle. The more you cycle through, the more the one in your arms will relax, the more you can deepen the connection and flow on your path.

The more you practice this, the more sensitive you will become to whatever tendency to move appears in those you hold. Transitory movements or aftereffects may come to the surface, or segments of the web of micro-movements that continue to play and bounce off each other. Be ready to support and follow whatever tendency appears.

Afterthought

Just as particle and wave in physics are two states of what is the same, the oneness in the emptiness at the bottom of the breath is the particle that, as a wave, rising up through our core, is the wholeness that engages our whole being. Once you feel that wholeness with someone in your arms, how can that love be anything but unconditional?

WATSU TRANSITION FLOW

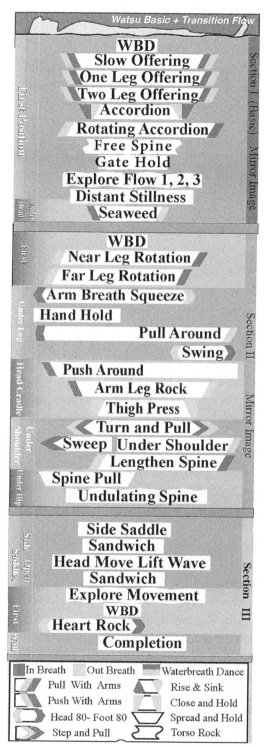

In Watsu 1, the simple moves introduced in Basic Watsu (16 hours) are followed by the complex breath-timed combinations and cradles of the Transition Flow (34 hours). In cradles we brace someone against our body with one arm, freeing our other arm to stretch and work with them. Typically, those who complete a course in Watsu 1, start practice sessions doing Basic moves on both sides, and the Transition Flow from the Near Leg Rotation to the Undulating Spine on both. The Side Saddle and the moves to the finish are done on one side.

The descriptions of the moves that follow are intended for the review of those who have learned from an authorized instructor how to adapt them without causing discomfort or injury.

In Watsu 2, the form learned in the Transition Flow is expanded with additional moves and stretches in each of its cradles. In the book that accompanies it, Watsu, *Professional Path,* greater detail is focused on adapting the form to whomever you have in your arms. Once you have thoroughly trained your body to be with someone in water by practicing the form over and over, you can leave the form behind and start learning the Free Flow of Watsu 3.

To increase stability, avoid jarring steps and create a continuous flow. All but two of the moves are done with our feet staying over the same places. Start out at a depth that allows you to settle down into the water with your legs spread as wide as is comfortable. Your foot someone's head is over is called the head foot. The other, the foot foot. Facing 80 degrees from center is called head 80 or foot 80. In the chart alongside, Watsu 1 moves done facing the head foot are under the head of the figure at the top, those facing the foot foot, on the other side.

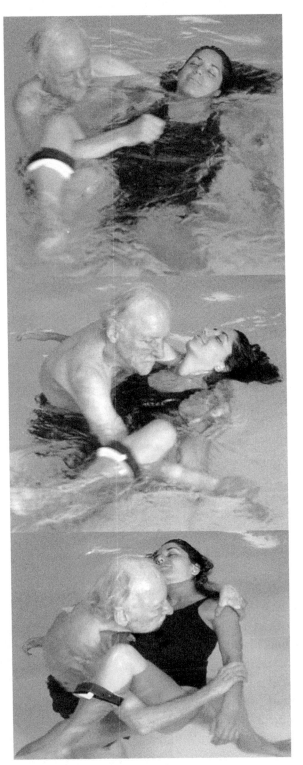

Near Leg Rotation

Completing the Basic moves on both sides brings you back to first position on Side A. Do the Waterbreath Dance. When ready, settle towards the foot foot on an outbreath. As you breathe in collect the back of their knee in your right elbow and rotate the leg up towards their left shoulder each time you breathe out. Drop back each time you breathe in, letting the water's resistance stretch the far leg. If necessary to protect your lower back, step your right foot back each time you drop back. Focus on the opening.

Far Leg Rotation

While rotating the near leg let go of it and, while continuing to turn towards the shoulder, scoop up the far leg. Rotate it to the same breath rhythm, pressing it towards the opposite shoulder as you breathe out, and stepping back with it as you breathe in. Focus on the closing movement. Explore stances from Head 40 to Head 80 and how a shifting of your weight forward can facilitate closings on the outbreath.

Arm Breath Squeeze

While rotating open the far leg, lower your shoulder deep enough to float the knee over it. Face Head 80. Hold the far arm with both hands, the left as high as possible. As you breathe in shift your weight over your head-foot. Each time you breathe out shift your weight back over your foot-foot (without pressing partner against you) as you squeeze the arm with your lower hand gradually increasing the squeeze as your own breath empties as if it were being squeezed out of your chest. Each time you breathe in, shift your weight forward and, maintaining a constant hold with your upper hand, slip your lower hand to squeeze a little further out the arm.

Alternatively, if the leg is too heavy to hold comfortably on your shoulder or too inflexible to hold in the upcoming Leg Cradle, pick up a noodle from the wall with your upper hand. Transfer it into your lower hand which centers it under the back of the knee. Continue with the Arm Breath Squeeze and the following:

Hand Hold

When you reach the hand, hold it with your thumb pressed in the middle.

Pull Around

Support the wrist. To maximize the sweep, twist back as far as is comfortable (Head120+). Pull the arm up and around, letting the head float into your hand and let go of the arm as partner continues to sweep around and out over your foot-foot, the knee sliding into your hand, the heel of your hand catching between the tendons in the back of the knee.

Alternatively, if using a noodle pull with it and hold it instead of the knee in the following moves.

Swing

The head is still held out in one hand, the back of the knee over the heel of the other hand. Stay low in the water in Foot 80, spine straight. Shift forward on each outbreath, partner swinging out in front of you. Shift back on each inbreath. Watch partner's arm. If it is about to bump against you, shift the side to which you hold your partner in front of you just enough to avoid the swinging arm's contact.

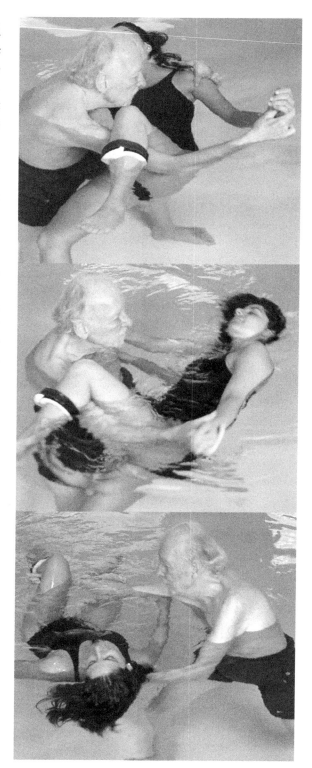

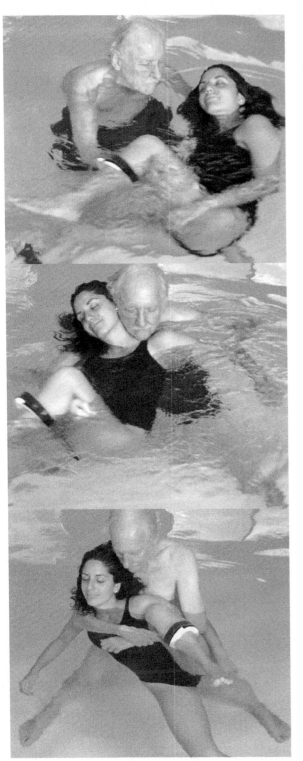

Push Around

When your partner just starts to swing back and is most on their side facing you, push the knee towards the chest causing their arm to come in front. Holding with arms straight, push partner around out over your head-foot to head 120. Without being pulled, the head passes in front of your face, the occiput arriving on the shoulder of the arm that had pushed, the neck comfortably propped against your neck.

Arm Leg Rock

As soon as the head arrives on your shoulder start pulling the leg back the other way with the heel of your hand that pushed it now hooked under the knee. During the pull the other hand can reach up under their back and make sure their head is comfortably positioned on your shoulder. Then it reaches up over the upper arm to pull it back. With each outbreath pull the leg toward the chest (a move that encourages outbreath), sweeping partner towards your foot-foot. With each inbreath pull the arm and sweep partner out over your head-foot. Avoid stressing your spine. Continue alternating the pull from side to side.

Thigh Press

Facing forward, pull the knee towards the chest. Reach over the shoulder with your other arm and slip it under the knee. Grasp its wrist with the hand that was first holding the knee. (Or grasp behind the knee with both hands). Stand tall and press the knee to the side of the chest without rounding partner's back. Hold.

Turn and Pull

One hand pulls the occiput (nested between thumb and finger, palm up) straight across in front of you as you take two or three steps, tractioning the spine. At the end of the pull slow down as your other hand pushes the hip to turn partner (without any torque or bending of the neck). When the turn is completed and partner is in front of you, switch hands under the head and pull to the other side. Repeat several times facing the same direction, dynamically slowing to turn and speeding up to pull.

Sweep Under Shoulder

When you come out from a turn over your foot-foot, instead of switching hands, flip the hand that is still under the occiput palm down and push the occiput cradling it between thumb and forefinger, the back of your forearm adding support to the upper back. As partner moves across in front of you, support the wrist and pull in a circle, cross-stepping forward with the foot-foot and back with the head-foot. Let go of the wrist and float the shoulder over your shoulder and support the occiput with your upper arm as your hand reaches under and around onto the heart center. Simultaneously reach under the far hip with the back of your lower hand and pull partner onto his side out over your foot-foot, bringing their jaw to your outstretched left forearm. Press against the top of the sacrum with the heel of your lower hand and, without pausing, continue onto next move.

Lengthening Spine

Stay low in Foot80. Keep partner on their side facing away from you. Without pressing the throat, keep your elbow raised under the head to keep it from falling back and straining the neck. Anchor your hand on the sternum while each time you breath in, the heel of your other hand gently pushes the sacrum down and out, lengthening the spine. Each time you breathe out, release the push of the spine generating a gentle wave.

If you have a good handhold on the sternum, instead of a wave, you can focus on lengthening, spreading your arms apart on each in breath.

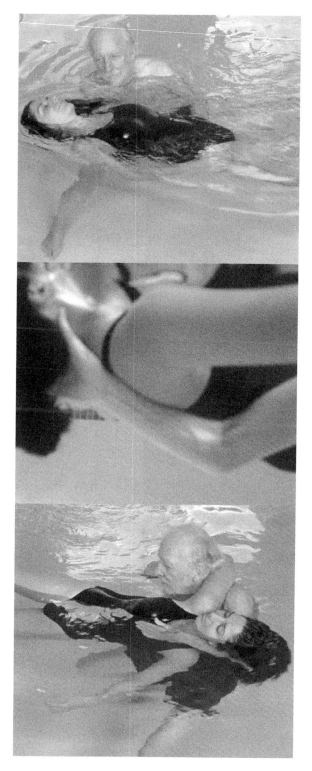

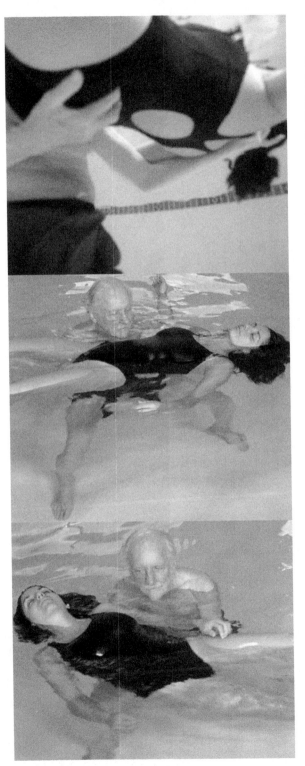

Spine Pull

Hold the occiput in the hand that was on the chest. Straighten that arm as you turn to pull partner out over your head-foot in Head80. With your other shoulder just under the hip, hook your fingers into the top of the sacrum. Settle back and pull to traction the spine. Hold.

Undulating Spine

Stay low. Stay under their balance point, palm up, fingers pointing to opposite side, your shoulder under their hip. Gently, rhythmically, lift. Keep your body suspended as you rapidly tap the bottom of the pool with the balls of your feet to encourage wavelike movements up partner's spine. Avoid jumping or jarring. Keep hand under the occiput open and still.

One Turn And Pull To Second Side

With your right hand push hip to turn him. When the head comes around the hand under it flips to push him in front of you where your other hand pulls his arm to sweep under shoulder. Do a mirror image of the above from side B. Hold the occiput in your right hand and pull partner as you slip your other arm under both knees to go into Side Saddle.

Side Saddle

Role partner's trunk up vertical as you lean back against the wall. If water is shallow enough, rest partner's head on your chest keeping both your feet on the ground, or brace your back against the wall, your right leg straight, your left foot propped over your knee or shin. Lower the backs of both knees over your upper left thigh (partner's hips dropping between your legs) and lean the side of the head against the right corner of your chest. Hold the cheek with your left hand and their shoulder with your right. Rest, doing nothing.

Sandwich

This saddle requires water shallow enough for you to be able to lower into it with spread bent legs over which you can support someone straddling your knees. If your partner might be uncomfortable with their legs open, skip this position. In Side Saddle lower the head into your elbow and, holding the upper back with your right hand, reach over or under and hold the far leg just above the knee. Lower your leg from under their left leg which is allowed to drop down to the inside of your right calf as you stand away from the wall. Step to the inside of that dropped leg catching its knee over your right knee as you lower into the water. If that doesn't happen easily, turn them towards their feet and step behind their near knee with your foot foot. Keep turning until their other knee comes to your right knee and you can easily step in. Place the other knee, which is still held in your left hand, over your left knee without forcing the legs apart. Partner's knees are out over your knees, maintaining space between you. The head lies on your right arm, facing you. Your right hand holds the upper back, its heel behind the scapula, while your left forearm presses from the front of the chest, between breast and shoulder. Keep this upper corner of the chest firmly sandwiched between hand and forearm. Keep the heel of your left hand lying gently over the jaw hinge, and your back straight and perpendicular to the pool bottom, as you shift your weight from side to side with each breath.

Head Lift

Switch partner's head to your left hand and with both hands hold your partner's head out in front of you. Settle down to engage your legs in lifting. Lift under occiput to lengthen neck. Hold. Without moving the head, slowly move your pelvis side to side.

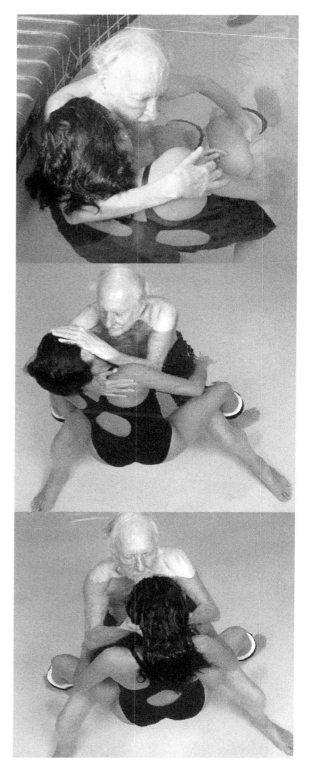

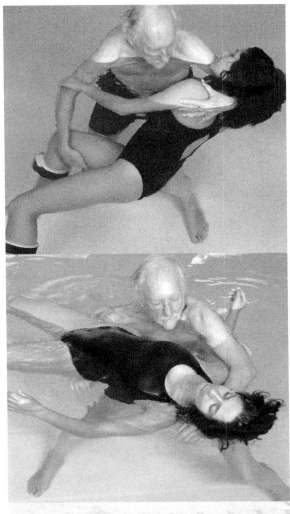

Sandwich 2

Place the weight of the head in the right hand, then lay the head on your upper left arm and mirror what was done with the head on the other arm. Overhold with your right hand and, holding close to the knee, lift the right leg to surface and return to the first position.

Explore Movement

Stay perfectly still. Notice whatever tendency to move is drawn out your arms from your heart. Let it draw you into a continuum that flows as your body, fully engaged, moves through new relationships of depth, distance and tempo, your feet being free to flow into new places without jarring steps. Throughout be careful to keep the head securely supported. Settle into the Water Breath Dance.

Heart Rock

Close to the wall, sinking to the foot foot, lower your right shoulder and with your hand slip the near leg over your shoulder. Face Head80. Gently place your right hand on the heart center and shift forward with each outbreath. If reaching under the leg would be awkward and/or they float, slip leg off your shoulder and reach over and place your hand on their heart center. Hold, rocking with the breath.

Close at wall.

Bring them to the wall to close as at the end of Basic Watsu.

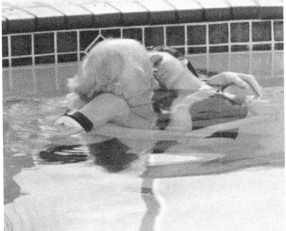

PRECAUTIONS

The Material in this book does not prepare you to work with medical problems. Occasionally you might have a friend or family member with a problem who asks to be watsued. Listed below are some of the more common precautions that Watsu Instructor and Physical Therapist, Peggy Schoedinger, has listed for aquatic therapists. Unless stated otherwise **don't Watsu anyone with these conditions.** *Don't Watsu anyone in water that is more than 98 degrees Fahrenheit. If in doubt about the safety of Watsu for a medical problem or impairment, don't proceed until you seek further medical advice.*

1. Fever, especially if over 100 F.
2. Cardiac failure, unstable angina, severely compromised cardiovascular system. Excessively high or low blood pressure.
3. Significantly limited vital capacity (below 1000 ml) and/or an inability to tolerate a 10% decrease in vital capacity.
4. Absence of cough reflex. Monitor extremely carefully.
5. Severe urinary tract infection
6. Unpredictable bowel incontinence
7. Significant open wounds and small open wounds on a person very susceptible to infection. It may be possible to cover a small, clean wound with a bio-occlucive dressing such a Tegaderm or OpSite.
8. Epilepsy, especially if uncontrolled. Light reflecting off water may increase probability of seizures.
9. Contagious water or air-borne infection/disease
10. Sensitivity to chemicals used in pool (chlorine, bromine etc.)
11. Severe peripheral arterial disease
12. Recent cerebral hemorrhage (wait until client is medically stable)
13. Uncontrolled diabetes (keep glucose tablets or juice available at pool)
14. Perforated eardrums. Keep water out of ears.
15. Kidney disease where patient cannot adjust to fluid loss
16. Patient with severely impaired ability to regulate body temperature
17. If patient is on long-term steroids or has had recent deep x-ray therapy, water tends to make already delicate skin even more fragile. Dry skin gently and thoroughly.
18. Uncapped tracheostomy
19. Deep vein thrombosis
20. Impaired sensation, especially in legs (stroke, brain injury, spinal cord injury, diabetes, peripheral neuropathy, etc.). Care must be taken to avoid client sustaining an abrasion injury on bottom or side of pool (a thin pair of socks can be very helpful in protecting the skin on the feet). Underwater lights generate considerable heat. Clients must not lean against them. Skin must be dried thoroughly after the session, especially between the toes. *(continued)*

21. Multiple sclerosis. Some clients are very sensitive to heat. Check first to see if your client tolerates warm weather, hot showers, etc. If heat is a problem, may need to do Watsu in a cooler pool.
22. Intravenous lines, heplocks, hickman lines etc. Check with physician.
23. Gastrostomies, colostomies, iliostomies, etc. can come into pool if the skin around the stoma is well healed. Drain bag first. Be sure to check seal before entering pool.
24. Catheters can usually come into the pool. Drain bag first. If possible, clamp catheter to prevent any reflux. Suprapubic catheters present a higher risk. Check with physician first.
25. Autonomic dysreflexia. Some clients with spinal cord injuries are susceptible to autonomic dysreflexia. This is a medical emergency which can cause the blood pressure to rise quickly. Watch for signs of autonomic dysreflexia (sudden severe headache, sudden increase in heart rate, sudden increase in blood pressure). Autonomic dysreflexia doesn't happen often, but when it does, it can quickly develop into a medical emergency. It is usually triggered by a noxious stimulus (distended bladder, increase/decrease in body temperature, etc.). Immediately determine the cause and remedy it. If symptoms worsen or don't improve soon, seek emergency medical help.

For more information see the chapter **Adapting Watsu for People with Special Needs** *by Peggy Schoedinger in* **Watsu Professional Path**

The New Watsu and Tantsu

By Minakshi

Having heard that Harold had developed both a new Basic Watsu and a course he claimed brought students back to the sources of Watsu, I welcomed his invitation to participate in them when they were offered one after the other on Long Island. From 1990 until I settled into my own Watsu center in Florida ten years later I had been in almost every class Harold taught at Harbin, first as a student and then as a co-teacher. The last class I taught with him was in 2007, so it was time for some continuing education. I also welcomed the opportunity to stay at Peter's beautiful Watsu center in Sag Harbor.

The new Basic Watsu's simpler progression allowed more time to focus on head support. Instead of being primarily presented for the experience, I saw the students in this Basic exploring a way of sharing Watsu with family and friends. I was also pleased with the ease with which the new Basic students took to an expanded Explore Movement.

Five of the Basic Watsu's ten students continued on into the following Watsu Tantsu Explore Flow course where they were joined by five students with a much wider range of experience in Watsu. Two were practitioners who had been practicing for a total of 25 years. And there was me with my twenty years of teaching. It was amazing how well we all worked together in this course's Explorer Teams and Rounds. We formed new teams of three each day that, since there were ten students, included Harold and myself. Each day we had a new theme to explore, such as how to incorporate a press, or how to bring our knees into play, themes that were simple but could be variously applied. After exploring with much feedback, the theme was introduced into the round in which each of us received a complete session from the other two. One started from our first side. The other continued from our second. Then both joined to conclude our session by watsuing us between them in what Harold calls a tandem float. I was as enthusiastic and inspired as the others and got as much out of it at the others. There is more to learn, before I will be ready to teach, so you will be seeing me assisting Harold with these classes again

I came to these courses to learn techniques to share with my students. But I got soooo much more. Before this class, I couldn't see myself teaching Tantsu. The second half of each of this course's six days was on land, exploring the newest form of the Tantsu that Harold started alongside Watsu to bring its nurturing holding back onto land. I observed how the land classes helped free up student's creativity for the water

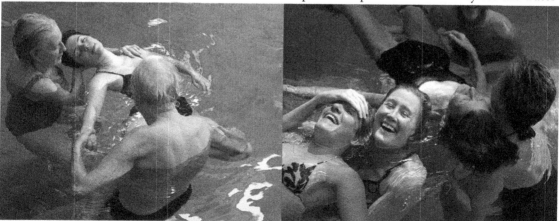

classes. Tantsu is introduced as a way to be with each other and not for learning new moves for clients. Its whole body containment helped us connect on a deeper level, both on land and in water. The safety we all experienced in that containment, helped us to truly "let go". Now, I want to learn more about creating the space for the "magic" that was palpably experienced by us all. I suspect it has something to do with the Tantsu class.

In the past, I had no interest in receiving from more than one person at a time. I am not good at multitasking. But what was happening in the Tandem Floats at the end of each person's session in a Round was something different. One time I was in the same team as Harold. The student floating my head in the tandem float freed Harold to move and stretch my legs in every way possible. Then he went into stillness with one hand on my hara and the other in the lower back, supporting it from below. I experienced the energy rising up my back. When it was my role to hold the head at the end of a round I could feel when the receiver's energy rose. Fascinated by my own experience, I watched what happened to others during that moment. I noticed how many of the students had a similar experience to me, but expressed it differently. Some got in touch with the love of their parents (they were receiving from a male and a female). One cried for the holding her grandparents never gave her but said they were good tears because now she knew how to hold them. Another cried over her abandonment as a child and realized she no longer had to carry the guilt for not being wanted. Another cried for joy. One woman said she got into the vortex down which the spirit enters into the womb and appreciated more than ever being a woman, having her own womb. It became obvious that whatever healing was "up" for people, could come to the surface in the tandem float's stillness of Hara Containment.

I see how this course can be a first step on what Harold calls the Explorer Path, and how it, and his new Tantsu, can bring the benefits of our work to a wider public, what Harold has always called the horizontal dimension. The vertical dimension, for professionals, has received a lot of attention up until now. Courses on this complementary Explorer Path are new electives for students becoming Watsu Practitioners on the professional path. I think it is wonderfully compatible and absolutely necessary for understanding the essence of Watsu. (It is not a sequence.) The icing on the cake, is that students can continue practicing these themes on their own, without a teacher. Hopefully, we will all find pools and the time to network with

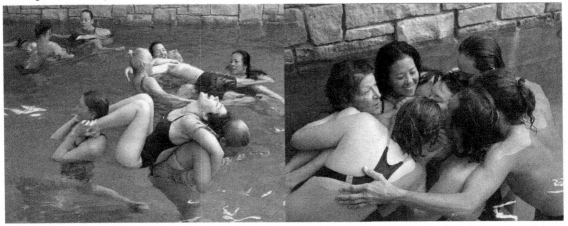

other practitioners to add a more full-bodied flavor to our practice. At the end of the course Harold asked how often students would want to join others on the Explorer Path if a pool was available. Their enthusiastic responses ranged from daily to twice a week.

Some students in our class shared:

1. As my introduction to Watsu, I felt very fortunate to learn Basic Watsu as well as the freedom to be creative. The first two days set the foundation. The Explore Flow class was extraordinary: the mix of people with different levels of knowledge was equalized. The experienced people provided many moves that were helpful for the new people and the new people provided non-traditional ideas and when these came together it was a magical playground in the water. The immediate feedback, encouragement and ideas from the receiver was invaluable. The highlights were the tandem "play".

2. I have taken Watsu 1. I took these classes because I love water and Watsu and to inform my acupuncture practice. The exploration sparked my creativity. I experience a happiness and freedom, I haven't felt for a long time. I learned about the heart chakra and connection to others on a deeper level. I had experiences of disappearing, death of the ego, and no self. I hugged my mom this week, when other times I cannot, because I have been so angry at her for years. I am going to hug my friends more

3. This is exactly what I needed to get out of my head and just be with the person. Even though I am very much a water person, I also absolutely love the coziness of Tantsu. When I arrived, I was terrified at the concept of explore flow. I was really hard on myself when I took Watsu 1 & 2. I am a perfectionist and was so preoccupied with perfecting all of the moves and sequences I felt really stressed and exhausted and inadequate. Now I feel so much more confident, creative and integrated.

4. I now feel confident that I can explore in professional sessions. Coming up with our own themes the last water session was fabulous. My partner's theme was "shoulder". Her exploration on me turned out to be an amazing shoulder treatment and made me realize that client requests can become themes to "explore" in sessions. This is a different than just trying to repeat all the moves that have been taught in a sequence that involves the shoulder.

5. I enjoyed the format of the themes and rounds. I would do another similar course anytime! I liked the tandem work. I am going to continue on this path because it is exactly what I was looking for: a way to deepen the connection with the people I work with, and bring the sacred aspect more alive in my practice—a way to connect heart to heart! Thank you

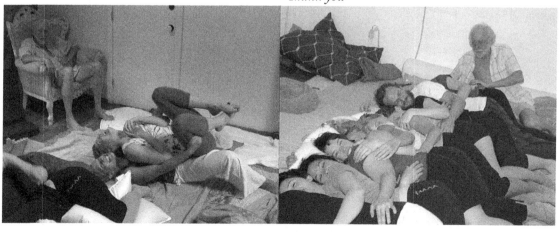

WATSU BASIC AND EXPLORER PATHS
POWER OF THREE MEETS THE POWER OF WATER

In the first use of triads in our Watsu classes, a third presented someone to the holder so that the holder could practice and learn a part of a long sequence before having to put it all together. The role of the third has evolved through the different forms developed for this book.

In the Explorer Team the third, without holding or touching, adds suggestions as to the different ways a theme or move could be applied. The closure from both sides in the Round that follows the team exploration, has evolved into Tandem Watsu.

In Tandem Watsu, the third usually focuses on supporting, balancing whatever the other is doing. If both are exploring freely it can be disturbing for the one held. In one on one Watsu Free Flow whatever is released usually takes them out around the pool. In Tandem Watsu, the support of the third creates containment and safety. Whatever is released can circulate within to wherever it is needed. At the end of a Tandem session it often finds its way up the spine which the two hold from each end.

A one on one Tantsuyoga was added to this book's second edition. In the third edition, having just developed a Tantsuyoga Round to accomodate more participants at a Yoga festival, the support of a third takes on a new role with their hand on the holder's back so that the holder could stay longer in their position on the floor, and go deeper into the breath with their eyes closed. This support has made Tantsuyoga accessible to many more people.

In the sixth edition, when I brought the movement as water, the ocean within, into Tantsuyoga, the third, up on their knees, their hands on our back, adds their own ocean within to our movement.

This seventh edition shows steps for anyone who has learned the Watsu Round to introduce it to two others at a time. This adds to our goal of making Watsu accessible to all.

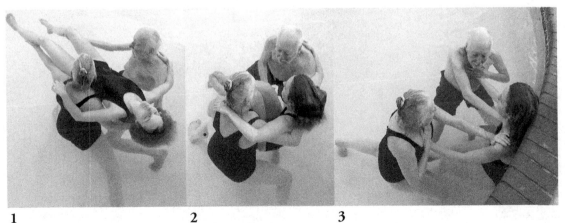

1   2   3

Watsu Round

In 2015, at a center in Mexico where children and pregnant women are regularly watsued, I developed a weekend for families that combined a round of three in water with Tantsuyoga on land. I called it Watsuyoga. The round worked so well that I decided to open all my beginning classes with it. In September, 2015, when the fire burned down Harbin Hot Springs where I started Watsu, we moved to Berkeley. I started looking for pools where I could continue developing Watsuyoga. With each triad staying on one side of the pool, I comfortably taught six in a pool just big enough for a single session. Since it is difficult to draw students who had never heard of Watsu to a weekend, I started teaching the Watsu Round in three modules, or Training Rounds, that were each complete in themselves. Each added additional Basic moves and ended with the same powerful Tandem Conclusion. Now, many Watsu instructors are finding the Watsu Round to be the best way to start their trainings.

In 2017 I was invited to offer a four hour Watsu Round at a hot springs in the Czech Republic during a conference on Watsu. Since there were more requests than the pool could accommodate, I was asked if I could divide up what I was offering. I offered the first training round in the pages that follow to absolute beginners and the second to those with some experience of Watsu. Both groups felt their experience was complete in itself. We are now training Watsu practitioners to offer the Watsu Round.

As I prepare this seventh edition I look over the stages in the earlier editions and see how much I attempt to put in words the experience and growth in awareness that led me to each stage. I have always prided myself in taking everything with a grain of salt, claiming that what I come to believe is based on my own experience. If this is true of others, how can I expect them to believe anything that they haven't experienced?

The obstacles in completely fulfilling the potential in Watsu is the shortage of warm pools and the difficulty in drawing people to something that seems so far outside their experience. I just read Blue World by the Marine biologist, Wallace Nichols, who studies the positive feelings brought up by being near, or in, water. Among the fondest memories that our body still carries is being in a warm bath, a memory that often includes others in the water with us, or watching over us. Presenting the Round as being complete in itself, a sharing of the joy we still carry from our earliest experiences in water, will probably draw more to the Watsu Rounds than any talk about energy or unconditional holding.

The five moves of the Tandem Conclusion are illustrated below by Minakshi, my daughter and myself. The individual basic moves can be seen in the Basic Watsu chapter.

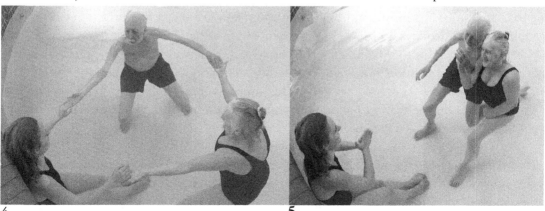

4   5

Bringing Others into the Watsu Round

When you have experienced the Watsu Round, you will want to invite your friends to join you in its next offering. If there is no next offering nearby, and you have access to a warm pool, instructions below will help you join and guide two friends through the Training Rounds. The moves are the same, but the instructions for training two from within a Round are different from those used by Presenters authorized to lead groups. Without an instructor to adjust the Holder's position and support from outside the three, Feedback, and helping each other, is vital.

Be the first Holder in each round's first two turns. Perform the basic moves in that role before you guide the one who, as Helper, had just watched you do them. Then be the Held in the third turn. There are three 90 minute Training Rounds that can be done separately. Each Round adds more Basic Moves. Each is introduced by:

1. **Waterchanics**: Join together in the water and explore how different our bodies, breathing and movement become when we are in water.
2. **Watsuchanics**: Practice the body mechanics underlying the basic moves we are about to learn as we imagine someone is in our arms.

In each turn, when someone has been brought from the wall, and that Round's Basic Moves have been done from both sides, the Tandem Conclusion, which is the same in all three training rounds, brings the one held back to the wall.

The text below in italics are instructions to you. All other words are to be memorized and spoken by you. Their intention is indicated by the indentation of the text:

Unindented text is spoken to both.

> Indented text that begins with (1) are directions spoken to the one being held.

>> Double indented text beginning with (2) is spoken to the one on the second side.

Training Round 1 The Waterbreath Dance

Enter the pool with the two others and have them imitate what you demonstrate.

Waterchanics

Explore with me how our body changes in warm water, how being immersed effects our breathing. Step into a part of the pool where the water is level with your navel. Stand as tall as you can, both arms out of the water, and focus on your breathing. Settle down, your legs spread to give you a wide base, your arms floating out in front of you, your chin just under the surface. Focus on your breathing. What differences do you feel from when you were standing taller... (buoyancy) ... Feel how that buoyancy adds to the lifting of your body each time you breathe in. Stand tall again. Notice the difference. Settle down again. Notice how the more settled you are, the water up to your chin, the more the water becomes a chair that supports your whole body, that rises with you each time you breathe in. Face one foot in warrior position, the arm out. Shift your weight forward without effort each time you breathe in.

Watsuchanics

Reach up. Find the base of your skull, a place where your hand fits. Hold your arms out. Imagine floating someone, one arm holding against the base of their skull, the other arm under the sacrum. Use the muscles in your arms to push them apart. Effort conveys tension to those in our arms.

Relax the muscles. Engage your whole body in keeping your arms gently pushed apart without tension. We call this tonus. It helps keep someone's spine lengthened and their neck protected when we float someone in our arms. Watsu is whole body. Stay a moment in the emptiness at the bottom of each breath. Feel how you are drawn up out of that emptiness each time you breathe in. You will be drawn up out of the emptiness again and again each time the one floating on your arms gets lighter as they breathe in. We call this the Waterbreath Dance.

We also use tonus in the closing. Stand facing each other. Imagine someone is floating between you, the one who is closest to me has their hand that is closest to the wall under the head of the one they hold. The other has that hand in their hand. Both have the receiver's calves in their other hands. Breathe in. As you both breathe out, in warrior position, shift your weight towards your foot foot, settle back to center and shift forward on each breath. Keep the head held and use tonus instead of force. Turn to face the head foot and, this time rock forward as you breathe out, your arms rolling their back up towards you, as your other hands, now under the thighs, push down.

The first time you float on someone's arms, reach up. Move the arm under your head to where the support feels best ... and the arm under your body. If you feel either arm efforting to lift you, gently lower that arm down. Once the support feels perfect, then close your eyes, Reach up again, without opening your eyes, anytime during the session, if you feel you can make the support more comfortable.

Preparation

Lean back against the wall where there are flotation cuffs.

(1) Whichever of you two has the least experience with bodywork or learning moves, stand to my left, your back at the wall (*referred to as female below*).

(2) Stand to her left. Hold her head with your right hand and lift up under her thigh with your left hand. When her feet come up to the surface, slip your hand, palm up, under her sacrum. Hold her. Her head is kept throughout about a foot from the wall, both ears in the water, her feet pointing to the center of the pool.

I check to see if her legs are locked. If they are, I gently lift up under them to unlock. If the legs are sinking, I take a float off the wall and slip it under the closest leg a couple inches up from the knee without closing it. If it pops that knee out of the water or the leg keeps sinking, I try another size float until the knee floats level with the surface. I close the first float and add and close a second float. I lift her ears out of the water and look at her:

(1) Keep your eyes open, I am moving into first position, your arm behind my back, my arms under your head and your balance point. Reach up and adjust them one at a time. When the support feels the most comfortable, close your eyes.

Basic Moves

I am in first position: her right arm under my arm behind my back, one arm under her head, my hand resting on her shoulder, my other arm, palm down, under the balance point, the place where her weight balances. I stay low in the water without lifting her up out of it. I keep her ears in the water.

(2) Reach out and hold her hara between your hands without applying any pressure, letting it move with the breath. Your hand nearest her head is underneath. Keep your

eyes open. When I close my eyes slip your hands away and stay connected to our breathing. Be brought up from the bottom of the breath each time we are.

Waterbreath Dance: I use all my senses to synchronize to her breathing and, once synchronized, I close my eyes. I rest in the emptiness at the bottom of each breath until the getting lighter of the one in my arms draws me up out of it. I repeat this several times.

I open my eyes and, looking at the Helper, slide my arm higher up under the head to make room for his arm.

(2)Enter into first position as Holder on side 2.

I am now in the role of Helper, starting out holding the hara between my hands and directing, as needed, the Holder on side 2.

(2)Do a mirror image of the Basic Moves.

Tandem Conclusion (numbered illustrations on page 42-43)

(2)Make sure the head is a foot from the wall and the feet point to the center of the pool.

I reach up under her shoulder and hold her head, not her neck, with my open hand in a way that will best support it during traction. In warrior position I reach down with my other hand and cup the belly of her calf.

(2)Reach under her shoulder and place your hand under my hand. With your other hand cup the belly of her calf.

Tandem Lunge-1: We look at each other and breathe in together. As we both breathe out, we turn towards her feet and, keeping her head fixed, shift forward to push her calves. We keep looking towards her feet. We stay in warrior and traction, lunging toward her feet on at least three out breaths.

Tandem Accordion-2: We keep our feet in the same place and pivot toward her head. We move our hands up under her thighs just above her knees. We make sure our forearm is behind her scapula. We look at each other and breathe in. On the out breath, we roll her back while our hands. On each out breath, we sink her hips deeper without bringing her knees out of the water, and, while keeping her head aligned, pull the back to bring her chest forward. When her chest is as close as it can comfortably come to her knees, hold the press at least three breaths.

Three Become One-3: We gently lean her back against the wall as we lower and spread her feet into a wide base. We place and keep the hands that lowered her legs on the corners of her chest. We lean her head against the wall. Anytime it is needed, the hand that is under my hand, can be brought out to adjust the head. Both hands that were under her head, lift up her hands. We look at each other and simultaneously hold her hands to our heart centers and close our eyes.

Opening the Circle-4: We open our eyes and, looking at each other, simultaneously move her hands away from our heart centers and raise our middle fingers up under the centers of her hands. As we open the circle, we press our other middle fingers into the center of each other's hands. We hold the circle open.

Namaste-5: We drop our fingers from under her hands and cross our arms that are nearest each other as our palms join in a Namaste. Our heads join behind to watch her open her eyes.

The two of us join the one at the wall to the same sides we started from. If this had been the first turn and there are two trainees, the one who had been held goes to the far left to present the one who had first started from the left to you. Otherwise the one on the left crosses over to your right where the one who just been held can present you to him in this last turn. xxxxxx

Training Round 2-the Offerings
Waterchanics

Settle in the Water. Breathe in. Breathe out settling down and staying a moment at the bottom of each breath in the Waterbreath Dance. On your next outbreath relax your right knee and slowly sink towards your right foot without rocking. Let the breath draw you back to center without rocking. Sink again. Keeping your feet in the same place, the next time the breath starts to rise, push against the bottom of the pool with your foot, causing your pelvis to turn towards the other side where your arm is out like this. Whenever you are ready to breathe out, settle down and, as you breathe in, push with your foot causing your pelvis to turn back to the other side, your other arm out to that side, your feet staying in one place but swiveling with each push. Continue. Feel how effortlessly movement and breath can be integrated in water. Notice how being in water helps you engage your whole body as you stay in tonus.

Watsuchanics

Imagine you are floating someone in the Waterbreath Dance, their head on your left arm. Sink to the bottom of the breath and be brought up to center through at least three breaths. The next time you breath out, relax your right knee enough to slowly sink to that side, to sink toward what we call our Foot Foot because it is the one on the same side as the feet of the one we float. Feel the potential of force in your bent knee. The next time you breathe in push against the bottom of the pool with your foot foot, causing your pelvis to turn and a vector of force arrive in your leading arm to pull the one in your arms around to the other side. Whenever you are ready, breathe out and settle down to the foot that will initiate your turn back to the other side as you breath in. Continue from side to side, keeping your whole body in tonus without compromising your alignment.

Preparation

The order of the three at the wall establishes the same roles as in the first Training Round.
    (1)If you needed floats, put them back on. Keep your eyes open until the support is best.
        (2)Present her to me.
I enter into first position
        (2)Hold the Hara from both sides until I close my eyes.

Basic Moves

Waterbreath Dance
Simple Offering: As I breathe out, I relax my knee enough to slowly sink toward my Foot Foot. I sink three times, letting the breath bring me back up to center each time without rocking. The third time I push against the bottom as I breathe in, causing her body to start turning. A vector of force rises up from that push into my leading arm that pulls her head around. Whenever I am ready to breathe out, I let her continue to float around while I settle into the Head Foot, that, when I breathe in, pushes to initiate the vector of force that arrives in the back of my hand to pull her hip.

I continue from side to side.

One Leg Offering: The third time my leading arm starts to pull her head, I leave my other arm where her leg can float over it. After I settle down to push from my head foot, my leading arm pulls her leg around. In both directions I maintain a continuous traction.

Two Leg Offering: The third time I pull the head, I notice when the far leg floats the closest. The next time I pull the head, I scoop up the far leg when it is the closest. I continue doing the Offerings three times with my arm underneath both legs applying the same mechanics and principles as before, maintaining a constant traction. After the third time I slip my arm under the balance point as I face center in first position.

I hold for three breaths and make room under the head for the second Holder's arm.

    (2)Enter into first position as Holder on side B.

I am now in the role of Helper, starting out holding the hara between my hands and directing, as needed, the Holder on side B.

    (2)Do a mirror image of all the Basic Moves.

Tandem Conclusion

We do the whole Tandem Finish as in the first Training Round

Training Round 3 Explore Flow
Waterchanics

There is continuous movement within our bodies. Stand as high out of the water as you can, arms straight out to the sides. Focus on whatever movement, whatever micro movements, there are within one arm ... and then within the other.

Drop down to your chin. Keep your feet in the same place. Hold both arms out in the water. Focus again on whatever movement there is within one arm ... and then within the other. Notice the difference when your arms are immersed. As you focus on the movement in one arm, notice if any movement in the other arm continues or balances that movement, or anywhere in your body. Notice how open your whole body is to movement in warm water. It is a continuum, movement that never stops, never repeats itself.

Block that movement to one side, holding your right arm bent at the elbow, as tight as you can. Your other arm stays out open. The movement of water within you is a river dammed up by your bent arm. Open that dam and let that river flow out your other arm, out through your whole body.

Watsuchanics

Stand and find on yourself major places that we will be holding. One is this hollow in the corner of the chest. The other is this hollow behind the hip. These are the places where the arms and legs first appear in the fetus. The arms are what we reach out to others with. We call these places the Heart Gates. Hold them. The legs connect us to the earth. We call these the Body Gates. Hold them.

You have someone's head on one arm. Your other arm is under their hips, clasping as firm as you can with the heel of your right hand pulling into the body gate on the other side, your shoulder pushing into the body gate on this side. Hold as firm as you can damming up the movement of the water within, the water within both of you. Your other hand is out under the head, open like this, ready to let whatever is released flow out your arm. Hold. Release. Flow freely with the river within. The hand reaching out under the head on your arm settles on the heart gate like this. The river within each of you joins into one river. Flow with it. Press with your right hand the near body gate as a fixed point, a rock that the river must find its way around on its way to the ocean, and it can't remain fixed long. The force of the river drives it, too, into the ocean. Now your two hands are holding the ocean between them, an ocean that moves in every direction. Reach across that ocean to the body gate on the other side. Enter into that one ocean. Become it.

Preparation
The order of the three at the wall establishes the same roles as in the first Training Round.
 (1) If you needed floats, put them back on. Keep your eyes open until the support is best.
  (2) Present her to me.
I enter into first position
  (2) Hold the Hara from both sides until I close my eyes.

Basic Moves
Water Breath Dance ... Simple Offering ... One Leg Offering ... Two Leg Offering

Gate Hold: When I return to center at the end of the Two Leg Offering, I clasp her Body Gates between the top of my shoulder or bicep and the heel of my hand reaching underneath. I support her head on my other arm, my hand out like this. If my arm didn't reach, I would place my shoulder above her hip. I hold as tight as I can without lifting her out of the water.

Explore Flow: I release the hold and let what was blocked flow out my arm and through my whole body as a river. I let her head move on my arm.

Heart Gate: I place the eminence at the base of my thumb in her Heart Gate, inviting the flow within her to join in the river.

Near Gate: I place the base of my other hand in her Body Gate as a fixed point, a rock in the river that everything flows around until the flow is so strong it pushes the rock into the ocean... Holding her heart gate and body gate, I am now holding the ocean between my hands, moving in every direction.

Far Gate: I reach over to hold her far gate, entering into, becoming the one ocean.

Stillness: I slowly lift my right arm and slip it back under the balance point in first position and return to the Water Breath Dance. After three breaths I slip my arm higher under her head to give you room to replce it.
  (2) Enter into first position as Holder on side B.
I am now in the role of Helper, starting out holding the hara between my hands and directing, as needed, the Holder on side B.
  (2) Do a mirror image of all the Basic Moves.

Tandem Conclusion
We do the whole Tandem Finish as in the first Training Round.

If they start every round with the same order at the wall, in each third turn, have the one who recieved present you to the one who was the last Helper (who is probably the most adept).

WATSU EXPLORER PATH

The Themes

Rather than a form such as the sequence of moves required to enter the positions on Watsu's practitioner path, those who share this path utilize a format, the steps to be followed when any three meet to explore together in a pool.

There are 12 stations laid out for your path in this book. At each you will be given a theme to bring to a Meeting, a move or position that has more than one way to be introduced into a session. Its description is kept short enough to be read at home and recalled when you join others in the pool without having to take the book along with you. The illustrations at each station are presented as suggestions and do not include all the possible applications of that station's theme. You may have learned some on other paths as part of a combination in a sequence. On this path explore them, and the principles they manifest, in a new way. Leave behind any concern about what can be done with clients. Explore what Watsu has for you.

Whenever you want bring a theme of your own invention to a Meeting, a theme that does not have only one way it can be done, or is part of a combination. Because each brings their own theme, students and practitioners at various levels of Watsu can meet and explore together anywhere in the world and nourish connection, continuum and creativity.

Each theme is explored first by the Team with the one being floated fully participating, adding suggestions and giving feedback. Then in the Round each receives a complete session in which the only feedback the receiver needs to give is what relates to maintaining their comfort. All they need to explore is how deeply they can surrender and receive.

The Flow

The Flow that follows the breath timed moves in this book's Basic Watsu was first developed as a way to lead into the themes in the Rounds on this path. Some themes extend the continuum established in that Explore Flow. Some, such as a press or a stretch, bring the flow to a still point. Some themes follow best if the arm is freed. Others if the holder stays in first position. Explore what is the best entry point with the Team before you introduce your theme in the Round.

The Side Change that follows each application of a theme can spontaneously lead us into another continnuum or still point, particularly if we keep our mind free as someone's other side arrives in front us. As the side change introduced at the first station brings that other side around, we are presented with arm, hip, leg, knee, foot, any one of which we can take hold of and continue the Explore Flow we were in on the other side. The more the flow is open to the spontaneous, the more our intuition and creativity is engaged, the deeper and longer lasting the effect can be.

Care

Though receivers accept the responsibility of monitoring their own comfort, adjusting their position and giving feedback, both giver and witness should still be looking for ways to improve and insure the best support possible is provided. If the receiver's legs tend to sink in a way that hyper extends and compresses their lower back, they should wear flotation cuffs, ones that float the knees just up to the surface without breaking through it.

Format

At each Meeting on the path the three share from two to three hours in the pool. There are three sections to a Meeting format:

Solo

On first entry into the pool each participant starts their solo exploration of how the water supports them and helps them surrender into a flow. Starting with the movements that underlie the opening moves, they continue on to whatever movements their station adds to their solo dance. If they arrive at a Meeting outside of class, one by one, without greeting, each can continue their solo dance until it is ten minutes past the hour set for the Meeting. Then each participant backs up towards the center of the pool and, leaning back against each other, support each other in a couple minutes of silence. Then they turn around and greet each other and, if it's the first time they meet, introduce themselves. They can discuss the options to apply to this meeting such as doing all the opening moves on both sides or starting the second side from Free Spine and whether to explore Tandem Moves in their Explorer Teams.

Explorer Team

For each Meeting in a class the instructor assigns the themes that students explore. Outside of classes each brings their own theme. During this section, which takes about thirty minutes, each explores all the possible applications of their theme with each of the others. Receivers give any feedback that might help the giver perfect his application of the theme. Witnesses add any suggestions that might come to mind during this section.

If the team agrees to explore tandem applications, the witness has a more active role exploring how best to support someone.

Round

The third section is a round in which each participant receives a complete thirty to forty minute session. The round has its own format that begins with Watsu Round's basic opening moves up to Stillness.

1. The first floater starts on side A with those opening moves. What follows this opening in a Tandem Round is described later. Otherwise the Stillness is followed with:

2. whatever variation of the first floater's theme enters into the flow

3. a side change to side B

4. whatever is spontaneously entered into

5. a second variation of the theme

6. a side change back to side A

7. whatever is spontaneously entered into

8. holding the receiver out in Distant Stillness.

9. While the first floater holds the receiver out in this stillness, the second floater, who had been witnessing everything through whatever resonances were awakened in his own body joins from side B in first position and continues as above, 1 to 8, exploring with his own theme.

9a. Alternatively, if time is limited, the second floater can gently hold the receiver's hara (abdomen) between his hands while he is being held out to him, connect to his breath within and then, in first position, start the above from Free Spine.

10. When the second floater arrives at Distant Stillness, the first, coming from side A, holds the hara between his hands.

11. The first floater explores all the ways his theme can be applied in a tandem while the second supports as needed.

12. Together they continue to the Tandem Mirroring and Finish introduced at Station 1.

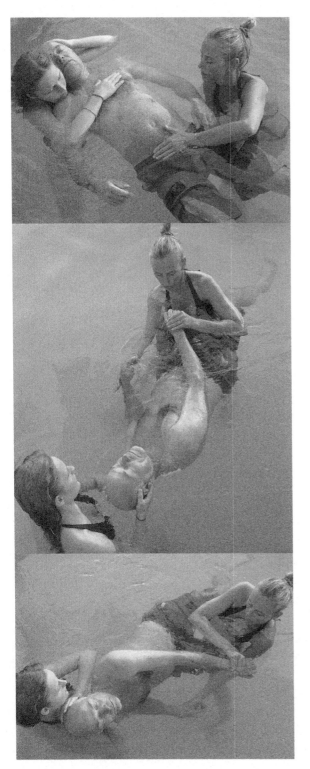

Explorer Tandem Watsu

We have always recognized Watsu's potential to help people access and share the joy in their hearts. We find that when Watsu is shared with more than one other it becomes even more joyful. Exploring as a team adds a creative playfulness to the path. Having two share in giving the complete session that each receives in a round, one from each side, and both together in a tandem float at the end, adds a new dimension.

The experience gained in learning how to explore and how to support in those few minutes of tandem floating that conclude each simple round, prepares someone for the rounds in Stations 11 and 12 where, after the opening moves on one side, the whole round is done in Tandem.

Containment

When we first started floating people in Watsu, we realized that holding accesses a level of healing beyond that of touch. Holding is the oldest form of healing, something a mother picking up a fallen child to hold to her heart knows instinctively. The value of holding has been corroborated in our Core Tantsu classes that introduce opening positions in which we cradle someone's whole body between our legs. Support at someone's base rather than triggering issues about intimacy adds to their sense of being contained. In containment people find safety. A new level of containment, a new dimension of Watsu, can be reached in tandem Watsu. The benefits and understanding that accompanies each of the Explorer's three roles merge into something greater than what is experienced in any one of the roles, into something even greater when the path moves between land and water. The wholeness that each experiences is a still further level of healing.

TANDEM FLOAT

Origins

Working in tandem first appeared in the Waterbreath Round that I developed in the early years of Watsu. Exercises that I later developed in which students learn new moves in groups of three turned out to be so successful that I decided to develop an Explorer Path on which everyone worked in triads. The course of its development and the discoveries made at each step appear throughout this book that required five editions to keep up with those developments.

When I saw how powerful Tandem Watsu can be, I developed a form for Watsu Practitioners that appears later in this book. Utilizing it with clients requires much practice and training. It also requires careful selection and preparation of the clients.

Explorer Watsu, Tantsuyoga, Tandem Watsu now appear in different combinations in watsu courses. Go to www.watsu.com.

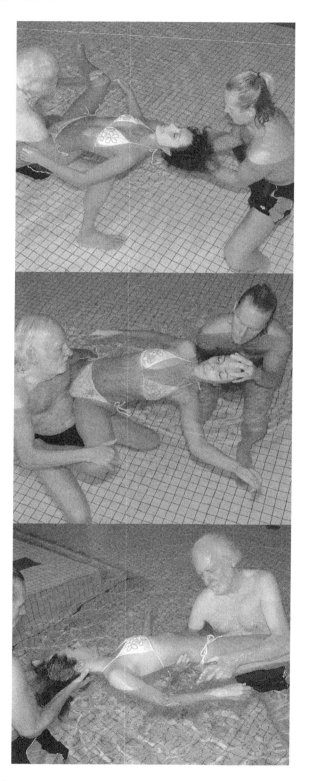

Station 1 Basic Elements

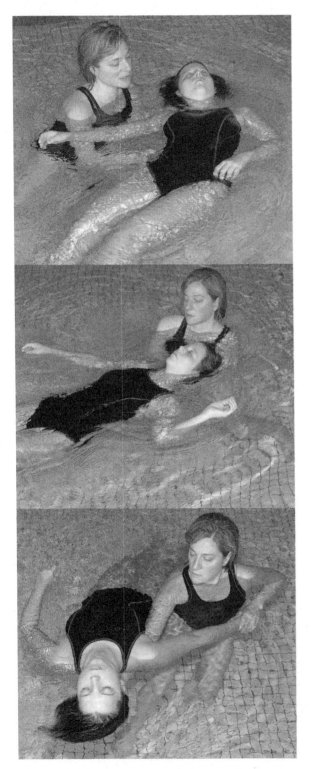

Every Round opens with the Opening Moves of Basic Watsu. has side changes that take the holder to the other side and back and concludes with the Tandem Mirroring and Finish. At this station the Team explores all these elements that follow the Opening Moves.

There are many ways to change sides. The one introduced at this stage is the simplest and brings the opposite side around to us in a way that presents many opportunities to explore. Those whose only previous training is Basic Watsu will find the more they use this Side Change the more opportunities they will find. Those who have learned other ways to change sides, can use them spontaneously.

Side Change

On side A in Free Float position we push against the hip until the other side of the floater comes around to us. Our feet stay in the same place. During the turn the head should be held and gently tractioned with an open left hand that keeps the neck and body in alignment. As the body comes around the right hand replaces the left under the head and the left is free to take hold of whatever comes around and explore entering into a continuum with it.

Tandem Mirroring

Both arrive in the first position, each from their own side, and share the support of the head and the balance point. In this mirror phase, the first floater mirrors every move of the second floater who initiates moves that can be mirrored and done together.

Tandem Finish

With the receiver's head close to the wall, join in a Waterbreath Dance, dropping together into the emptiness where the breath lifts you as three become one. Finish as in the Watsu Round or hold the knees from each side. Raise the head as you lower the hips. Spread the knees and place the feet into a wide base as you lean the back against the wall. Each gently presses a shoulder to the wall with the hand that lowered the knee while their other hand holds the receiver's hand to their heart. Hold. Simultaneously move back supporting the hand that was at your heart with your middle finger while your other hands hold each other to make a circle. Release and step back. The receiver presents, from side B, the one in his right hand to the one in his left to start the next turn.

Team

The witness holds someone out from side B. Enter first position from Side A. Overgrip the near leg. Explore with Free Arm. Once the arm is freed bring Side B around to you with the Side Change. Explore with whatever spontaneously comes to you. Return to Side A with the Side Change and Explore. Hold the receiver out in Distance Stillness to the second floater, who does the same as above from that side and back and holds the receiver out to you. Join from Side A, and, holding the receiver between you, mirror whatever the one on side B does. Continue with the Tandem Finish. The one at the wall presents, from side B, the one who had been in his right hand.

Round

FIRST FLOATER: Follow the opening moves with the Side Change to B and back, exploring the spontaneous continuum on each side. Then hold them out in Distance Stillness.

SECOND: Repeat above from side B.

BOTH: Do Tandem Mirroring (led from side B) and the Tandem Finish.

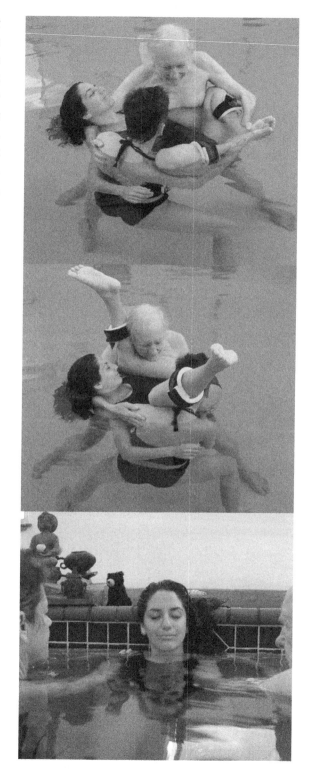

Station 2 Breath Shift

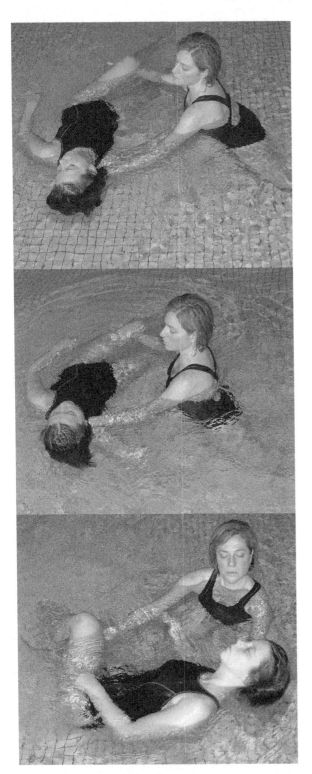

Stance

Up to now, except for the offerings, most of our stances have been center facing. In most our feet stay in the same place. In the 360 circle of directions that surround us we can mark the point in front of us as 0. Keeping the balls of our feet in the same places we can turn a little more than 120 degrees to either side. A turn of 80 degrees takes us into a stance called the warrior position. This is a very useful stance in Watsu. We call it an eighty, further defining, when needed, which side we turn to in relation to the one we float, Head 80 or Foot 80. Our feet and core face that direction.

Breath Shift

Facing 80 degrees to one side in water with our feet separated as far apart as is comfortable, we can shift our weight from one foot to the other with great ease, coordinating the shift to our inbreath and outbreath. Holding someone there are many moves we can coordinate with the shifting. If it is a move pressing into the body or some part of it, we usually breathe out as we shift forward. If it is a move in which some effort is put into lifting, we usually breathe in. If it is a move in which we pull towards us, we usually breathe out as we pull. In every case both feet stay over the same places, the heel of the foot in back rising as you shift forward.

Solo

Follow your opening dance with exploring the Breath Shift. Turn 90 degrees to one side. Notice how difficult it is to maintain your balance when your feet are pointing down the same imaginary line. Turn back 10 degrees. Notice how easy it is to maintain your balance in an eighty. Staying low in the water shift back and forth always changing direction just before an effort would be required to send you back the other way. Hold your arms out to push and shift forward as you breathe out. Add a lifting effort to your arms and shift forward as you breathe in. Hold your arms out to pull and shift back as you breathe out. Explore turning from one eighty to the other while keeping your feet in the same place.

Team

Explore, with much feedback, different ways to hold someone in an 80 and swing them out as you breathe in … and ways to gently press into them as you breathe out … and ways to hook and pull as you shift back breathing out.

Explore ways you might bring a breath shift into a Tandem Float, both when one supports and when one mirrors breath shifting together, towards the head, with the legs straightened out or over their shoulders, and towards the hips.

Round

FIRST FLOATER: Follow the Opening and four stage Explore Flow with whatever breath shift move it most naturally flows into. Continue with the side change, the spontaneous, a second breath shift move, the side change back and the spontaneous that take you to Free Float Stillness.

SECOND: Repeat above from side B.

BOTH: After connecting to Hara, First introduce moves that utilize breath shifting while Second supports. Then Second introduces moves that First can mirror.

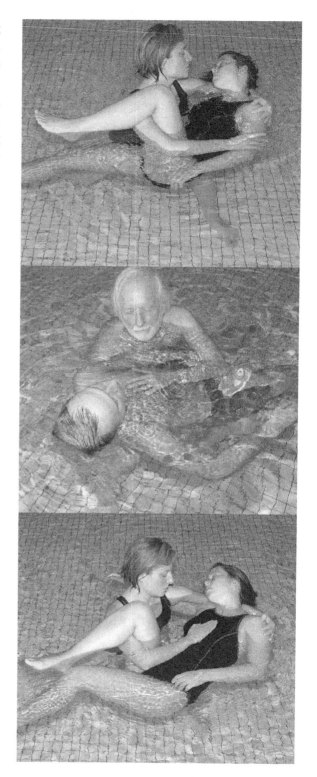

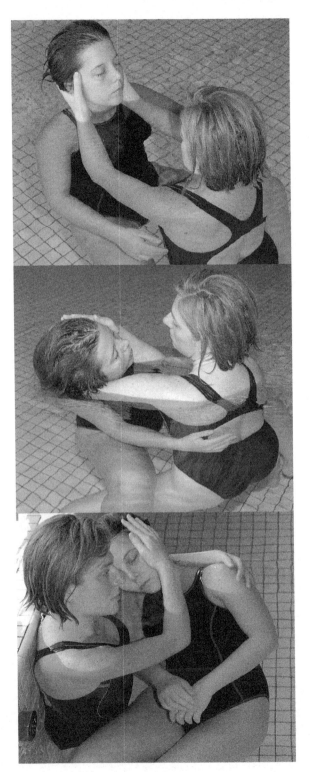

Station 3 Saddles

Opportunities

There are some positions that present so many opportunities that it is difficult to just flow through them, passing them all up. Satisfy your desire to explore everything you can do in a saddle while you are in the team. Wait for the moment you have someone in a Saddle in a Round to flow into whatever move first comes to you.

Saddles

A Saddle is when someone is sitting on our legs, usually facing us. The Saddle that provides the greatest access to their body, and consequently the most opportunities, is the Open Saddle in which someone's legs are open as they straddle both our legs. Keeping them held out close to your knees lessens any discomfort that might arise because of its closeness. If it does, explore some other way to put them into a saddle without opening their legs.

Solo

Follow your opening dance with finding the perfect depth for a saddle, a depth where you can feel you are sitting in the water with your thighs out at right angles to your torso. Explore moving in that position, keeping yourself balanced with the help of the water.

Team

Explore different ways to get someone into an open saddle facing you. Explore the full range of moves that can be done in this position with feedback accompanying each. Explore how the open saddle can be used as a side change to the other side. Explore how instead of opening their legs you can have both legs sitting over your thigh or both legs clasped between your thighs as you work with their body.

Explore saddles in a Tandem. First can come between the legs as Second lifts Third up into the Open Saddle from behind and Both explore how they can coordinate their moves from front and back. Second can pull Third's knees to his chest while First turns and backs under them becoming the supporter while Second explores what can done in this Back Saddle and then lifts and lowers Third out of it. Explore other saddles in Tandem.

Round

FIRST FLOATER: Do the Opening and the four stage Explore Flow. Flow into a saddle and, after doing a move in it, cross to the other side where the spontaneous waits for you. Follow it with a different Saddle or a different move in the same. Continue back to side A and the spontaneous and conclude with Free Float Stillness.

SECOND: Repeat above from side B.

BOTH: Introduce saddles into a Tandem Float.

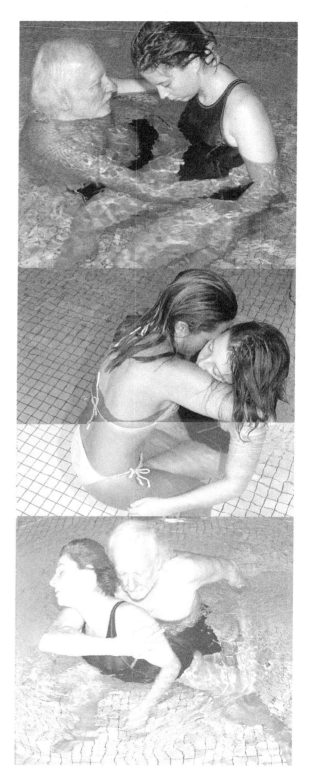

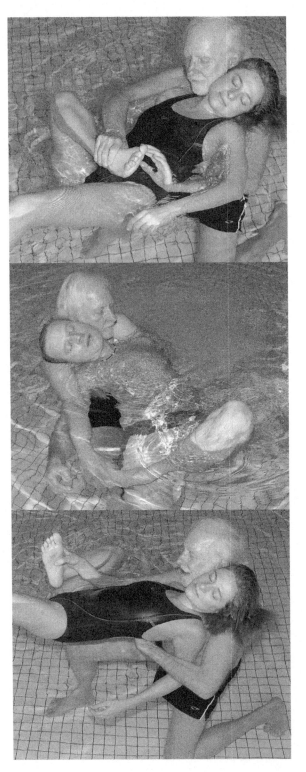

Station 4 Cradles

Holding

Watsu's holding, cradling someone in our arms as we float and work with them, has always been recognized as a key to Watsu's power to heal the wounds of separation. The kind of holding in both Watsu and Tantsu is a containment within which is safety. Rather than mothering or infantilizing the one in our arms our holding helps them recover whatever base of love may have been established the first time they were ever held.

Cradle

A Watsu Cradle is a position in which we cradle someone between our body and arm in a way that frees our other arm to explore. A simple cradle we can sometimes use as a side change is to press either leg to their chest and pull their back around up against our chest. As long as we can comfortably keep the leg pressed to their chest with one arm and their head supported, we can explore what our other arm can do with them.

Solo

Follow your opening dance with pulling up one leg at a time to the side of your chest with your elbow under your knee. Explore what pressure feels best and how to balance in this position.

Team

Explore pulling someone's far leg to their chest and moving their back up to your chest, their head on the same shoulder your arm is coming out from to hold their leg. Explore what your other hand can do with them in a cradle. Explore likewise with a near leg cradle, pulling their near leg to their chest. Be careful to keep the nose out,

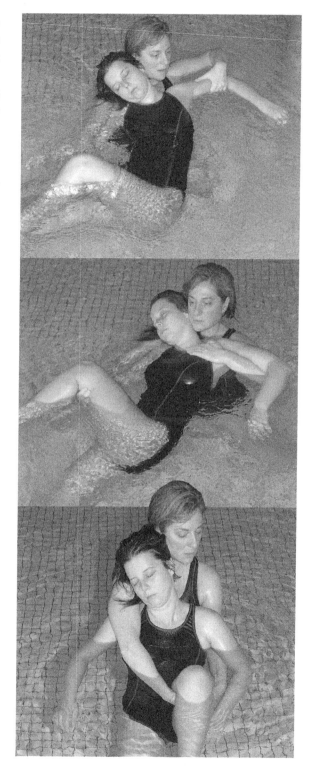

the head supported and the neck comfortable. Give copious feedback. Avoid any twisting of the back when it is curved. Explore ways to come out on the other side from this position.

In Tandem explore cradles and what can be done with them in both support and mirror modes.

Round

FIRST FLOATER: Do the Opening and four stage Explore Flow. Flow into a cradle with either one of the legs and explore how it can take you to the other side, exploring whatever comes to you mid-side change. After coming out on the other side into spontaneous moves, return with a different cradle and mid-side change exploration. After coming out into spontaneous moves, conclude in Free Float Stillness.

SECOND: Repeat above from side B.

BOTH: Introduce cradles into both supported and mirrored tandem floats.

Complete Format

Station 2 presented the complete format of the round: breath moves, stillness, explore flow, one application of the station's theme, a side change, a spontaneous move, another application of the theme, a side change back, another spontaneous move, free float stillness and, after both floaters have completed their side, a Tandem Float with both supported and mirrored phases. This format is followed in the rest of the stations. In this station and some to follow the application of the theme may itself be a side change. Each theme will only appear one time at the theme's place in the station introducing it. It may return in the spontaneous moves that follow side changes in subsequent sessions.

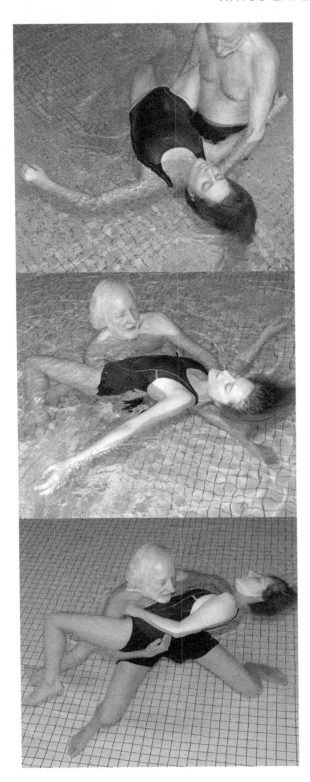

Station 5 Overgrip

Overgripping

An overgrip, reaching over with an arm, was first introduced in the third phase of Explore Flow. At this station we explore the opportunities overgripping one or both legs present as well as overgripping a thigh.

Explore Flow 5

A fifth stage of Explore Flow can be added to the Basic moves that open a session in a round. In the fourth stage you reach over to the body gate and explore how the flow initiated in the earlier stages can continue while reaching over. In this fifth stage explore further what movement accompanies their body's being repositioned against yours. Explore wrapping your right arm around their buttock as your right hand, pressing the muscle in the lumbar, carries the flow into a wave up their back. Explore how your left arm against the shoulder can send whatever wave comes up back down the back. Reaching up under their back, explore how the head can be floated into your left hand and how, when your left arm holds their head out straight, the new way their body is engaged against your side affects the flow. If their body comes to rest on your leg, explore how that point of contact can become a fulcrum around which the flow continue. Continue as one variation of your theme enters the flow on your way to a side change.

Dolphin Wave

If their thighs are not too wide and your arm is long enough, reaching around both legs just above the knee your hand can curl up under their lower leg far enough to be able to both push and pull that leg in a way that generates a wave up their back. Being in Position 1 with your arm supporting the occiput, your other hand can push the wave back down their back. Keep your own body far enough from theirs to avoid blocking the wave. When the wave is complete you can pull the overgripped legs and upper back to hold them tractioned and wrapped around you, hara to hara.

Solo

Follow your opening dance with exploring movements with your arms and the wave in your own body.

Team

If you can overgrip both legs far enough, explore the Dolphin Wave. Explore other ways to use an overgrip. Explore overgripping the near thigh to reach under and hug and work the near hip, to hook the sacrum and traction, and to work the far hip. Explore other ways to initiate a wave.

Explore overgrips that can be brought into both supported and mirrored tandem floats. While Second supports the head, First wraps his arm around the thigh holding the hip, his other hand on the hara. Explore other ways to bring a wave into their body.

Round

FIRST FLOATER: Follow the Opening and the five stage Explore Flow with whatever overgrip move best enters the flow. Follow the side change and the spontaneous with another overgrip move. Continue your flow back to Stillness.

SECOND: Repeat above from side B.

BOTH: Introduce overgrips and waves into a tandem float.

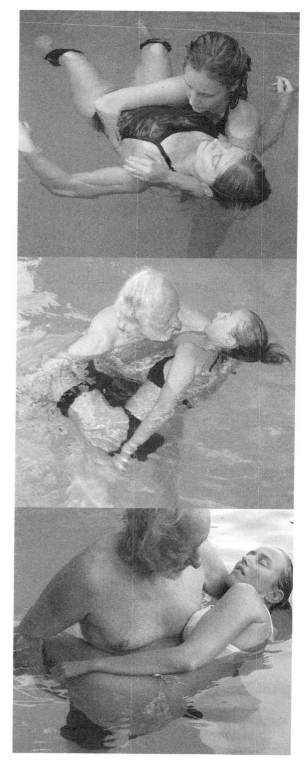

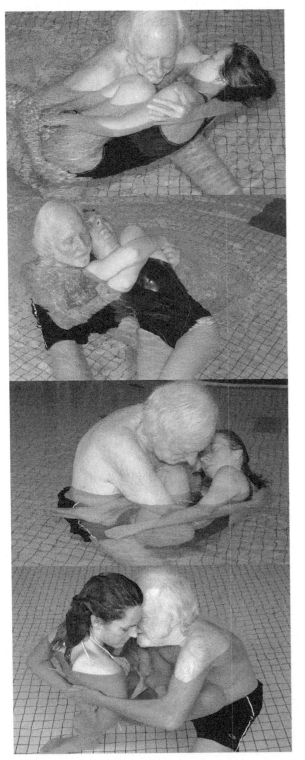

Station 6 Presses

Hold and Release

In presses we tighten our hold of someone between two parts of our body. This can be followed by a release, a moment of expansion, of feeling the body without boundaries, something enhanced by being in water. A release of a press can be accompanied by a moment of stillness, of listening for whatever inner movement may be being drawn up into the newly opened space.

Presses

Before the first stage of Explore Flow we introduced on optional press, holding someone's body gates between our shoulder and hand. Other times you will find yourself in a position squeezing someone's shoulders between your chest and arm. The most common press is pressing either leg to the chest. A leg press can be accompanied by shifting forward and back with the breath as you face eighty degrees to one side. Keep the memory of the Breath Shift in your body and let it come into play whenever a move can be enhanced by it.

Solo

Follow your opening dance with exploring ways to contain yourself in a press. Facing in an eighty cross your arms to clasp your shoulders. Tighten the clasp as you shift back breathing out. Each time you shift forward open your arms as you breathe in.

Team

Explore with each person ways to fold one or the other leg between you and press its calf to your chest. Notice how this can open their lumber, an area you can pull into with your hand. Notice how you can amplify that pull by shifting forward and back in a head or foot eighty position. With copious feedback explore what pressure each prefers and how to keep their back straight and their neck (and yourself) comfortable. Explore with each leg. Explore with both an overgrip and an undergrip. Explore other ways to hold them in a Press and when possible, ways to integrate breath shifting.

Explore presses in a Tandem Float. Explore ways to hold someone pressed between you and ways to coordinate simultaneous presses such as that of the shoulders and hips. Explore ways to release the press into expansions, pulling apart.

Round

FIRST FLOATER: Do the Opening and the Explore Flow. Bring a press into the flow. Follow the side change with a different press before continuing your flow back to Stillness.

SECOND: Repeat above from side B.

BOTH: Introduce presses into a Tandem.

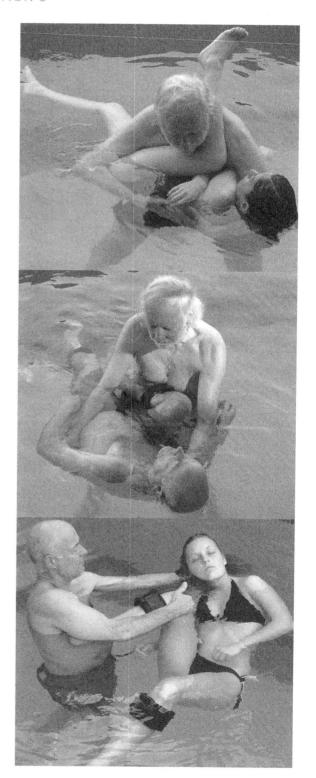

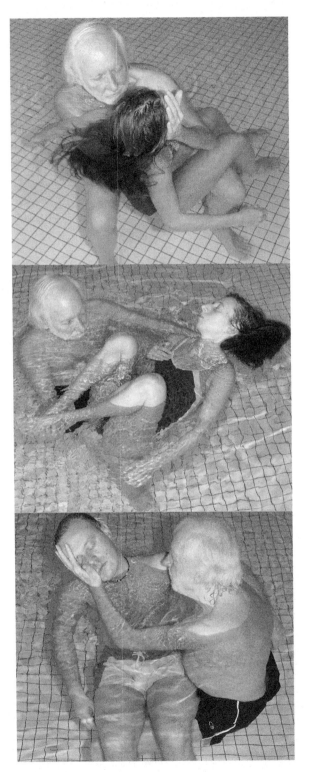

Station 7 Accordions

Compression and Expansion

Bringing both knees to the chest compresses and pushes air out of the lungs at the same time as it lengthens the spine. As we bring the knees back out the lungs expand drawing the air back in. When the knees are pressed to the chest don't wait for them to breathe because they may be waiting for you to open. You can start opening as they breathe in or closing as they breathe out, but once started continue to the rhythm of your own breath that you synchronized to theirs earlier. Feel the expansion of your own body. Keep their neck aligned with their spine. Tractioning the occiput through both phases helps prevent hyper extension of their neck.

Accordions

The most common accordion is executed in Position 1 with both knees over your arms. As you press the knees drop the hips into a sitting position and traction the neck. A Leg Accordion can be executed when you have both knees on one thigh and your arm reaches up their back under their near arm. Stay low and balanced in the water as your thigh presses their knees towards their chest and your forearm pushes their back and your hand keeps their head aligned. Your other hand, if your arm is long enough, can reach around to add to the pull of their back or it can lightly hold the face. If the water is shallow enough, or you have a step to prop your foot on, instead of raising your thigh all the closing can be done with your forearm behind their back. A Wall Accordion can be done pressing into their back with your chest as both feet are propped against the wall, your arms reach between their knees to hold their shins.

Solo

Follow your opening dance with exploring expansion and contraction as you move around the pool.

Team

Focus on forms of the Leg Accordion with copious feedback on rhythm, pressure and support of the head. Explore different uses and placements of the hand that has not come from behind the back to support the head. The Leg Accordion cannot be safely executed from Position 1 when our arm is over their arm. Our arm has to come up under their arm to be able to press into the back and support the head at the same time. Explore the Wall Accordion keeping them aligned and their head supported with your chest as you shift your weight against their back.

Explore tandem accordions. While Second supports the head, First lifts and props the knees over his shoulders. Explore. Holding the hips from both sides initiate a slow seaweed swaying of their body. Holding under their hips initiate a wave up their spine. Second can explore supporting the head with his chest as he pulls both arms up over his shoulders. Explore other moves with the arms. Explore ways to bring their chest up towards their knees and accordion them between you. Supine again First lowers and spreads the legs and hara to base works their hara.

Round

FIRST FLOATER: Follow Opening and Explore Flow with an accordion. Follow Crossing and Spontaneous with a different accordion. Continue your flow back to Stillness.

SECOND: Repeat above from side B.

BOTH: Introduce accordions in Tandem Float.

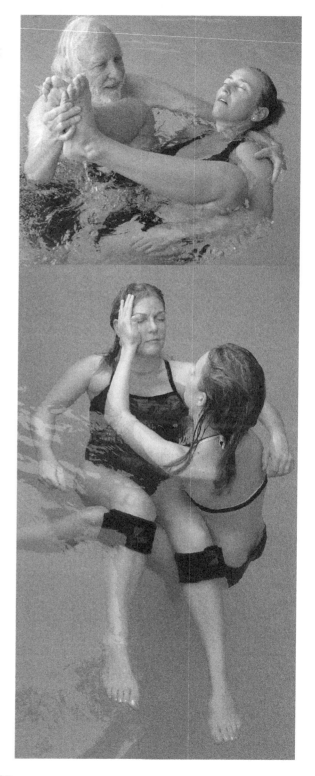

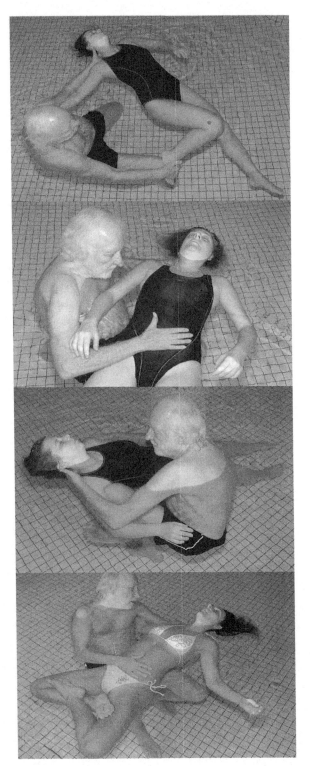

Station 8 Knee and Foot

Pressure, Support and Fulcrum

Bringing a knee or foot into play introduces a third element when someone is floating on our two arms or hands. It can be brought up to press into or massage a muscle. It can be brought up as a support or as a fulcrum to stretch or move the body around. They are free agents that can be invited in anytime during a session.

Knee and Foot

The knee is more versatile than the foot. The foot can come into play when we are holding someone out from us and is usually used to push. The knee can be raised in more positions. The knee's rounded surface invites pulling or rolling parts of the body over it. You may feel someone's body calling your knee to it. Answer that call.

Solo

Follow your opening dance with exploring the water's support by contrasting its complete support with a partial support. Stand close enough to a wall of the pool that you can reach out and lean lightly against the wall. Notice where there is a fulcrum where your weight and its support is centered between your feet on the bottom and your hand against the wall. Remove your hand from the wall and settle back into the water. Notice how peripheral the support becomes, your body being supported from all sides by the water.

Explore how if you reach out with one arm some part of your body moves or shifts to keep you balanced. Reach out both arms and, keeping your feet in the same place, turn with the breath from side to side. Notice the slight but still dynamic balancing that accompanies your turning with your arms out. Slowly lift one foot and notice how your body rocks slowly back to balance that move, and slowly rocks forward to return your foot to the floor without effort. Explore how a shift back can raise your foot. Explore a water walk that moves you around the pool just by shifting your weight effortlessly.

Team

Explore floating someone in front of you as you raise a knee and pull or roll different areas of their body over it. How does the effect change when you hold their knee or foot in your hand. If you bring your knee up into their lower back be sure to apply pressure towards their sacrum to traction their spine. Can you roll their Hara gently over their knee. Get feedback. Explore supporting up under their armpit with one knee while pressing the other side of their chest towards that knee. Explore pulling their gluteus or the bottom of their foot over your knee. Explore supporting them on one knee while changing positions. Explore using a foot.

Explore using knee or foot in a Tandem Float. While Second continues supporting the head and the balance point, explore integrating your knee into work with both hands. Move to the feet as Second moves up under the head and continue exploring. Roll both feet down over your knees.

Round

FIRST FLOATER: Do the Opening and Explore Flow. Without interrupting the flow and without exploring all the possible uses of the foot and knee, incorporate whatever use best fits into the continuum. Follow the side change and the spontaneous with one other way to work with your knee or foot. Continue your flow back to Stillness.

SECOND: Repeat above from side B.

BOTH: Introduce knee and foot in Tandem.

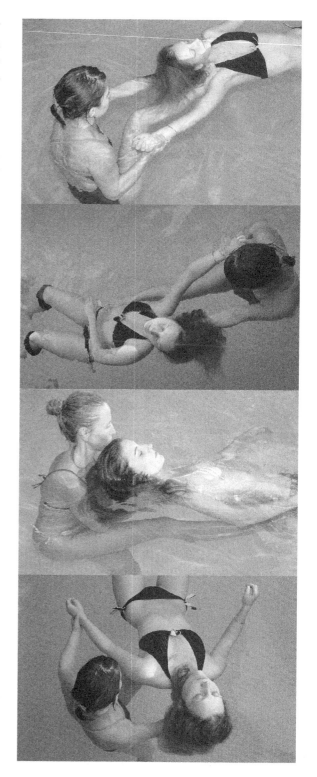

Station 9 Wall and Steps

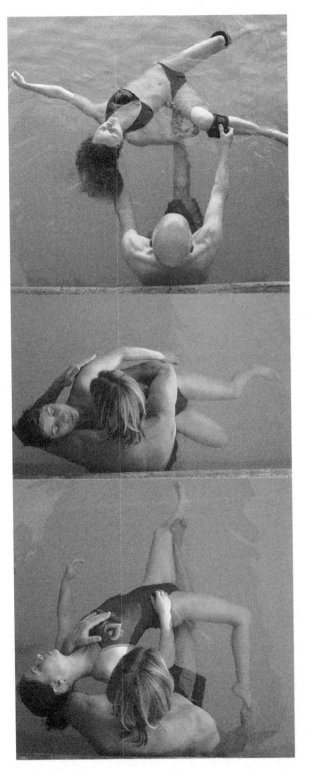

The Wall

The most common use of a wall is for support, usually with our back against it. This frees one leg to reach out and support or work with the knee or foot when someone is floating out in front of us, their head on our shoulder. Alternatively the freed leg propped on our supporting leg or against the wall can support someone seated on or straddling our thigh. They can be facing away, to the side or towards us. Most positions at a wall frees our hands to work with greater focus and depth than when someone is floating.

Steps

The usefulness of steps depends on their configuration. If there is a wall alongside the steps and the steps are wide enough we can lean back against the wall with our feet out on the steps as we hold someone. Without a wall some steps can be used to sit and lean back on as your feet can press against the sacrum of someone floating out in front of you. Steps can also be used to raise a bent leg to improve the support for some moves.

Solo

Follow your opening dance with explorations of movement when part of you is touching or leaning against the wall or the steps.

Team

Explore what each can do with their back at the wall. Explore what they can do with their knee or foot while holding someone out in front of them. Explore what can be done settling someone down on a thigh raised and propped against the wall or the other leg. Explore with them facing away, facing to the side, and facing you straddling your leg with copious feedback.

Explore how the wall or steps can be used in the Tandem Float.

Round

FIRST FLOATER: Do the Opening and Explore Flow that leads into a way to work with the wall. Do whatever side change, spontaneous, work at the wall, side change back and moves come into the Flow. Conclude in Free Float.

SECOND: Repeat above from side B.

BOTH: Introduce a way to use the wall or the steps while floating someone together.

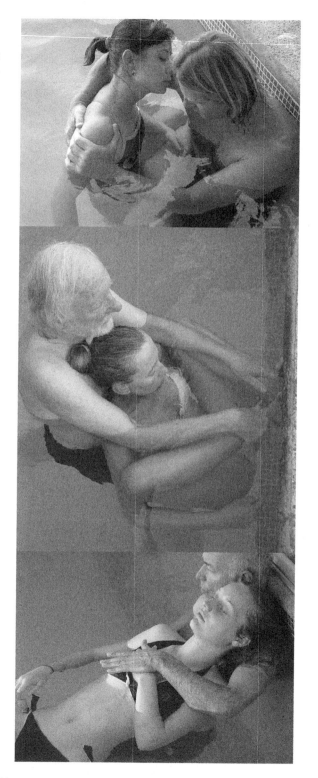

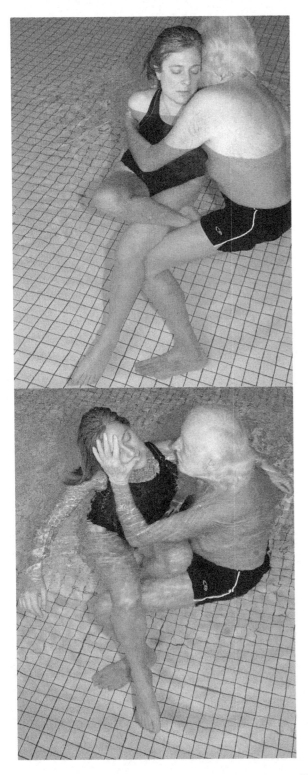

Station 10 Catches

Using our own body

In holds, presses and catches your own body becomes a platform to support all or a part of someone's body. In the second stage of Explore Flow the side of your body can incidentally stretch the arm back. Maintain awareness in your whole body of whatever effect any contact might be having. When Both are floating in the round explore being there as a double platform.

Catches

A catch is a little cousin to a press. Rather than a whole leg you usually capture a foot against some part of your body while someone is floating in front of you. The most used catch is when someone's far leg is pulled over their near leg, their foot protruding enough to hook it against your body, usually at your thigh. Another catch is keeping a heel pressed towards the buttocks by propping someone's foot on your thigh. A different kind of catch is when the feet are caught across someone's own legs as in Lotus. Positions in which you have someone wrapped around your waist could also be considered a catch

Solo

Follow your opening dance exploring movement on one leg with the other foot propped over your thigh or held in your elbow or with its heel pressed to your buttock. If you can comfortably get into lotus, float in lotus with your arms up over your head.

STATION 10

Team

Explore catches with the foot of the far leg pulled far enough over their near leg to hold it caught against your body. Explore the range of places on your body where you can catch it and how their back may need to be held pulled or rocked to keep from losing the catch. Explore the access it provides into their lumbar. Explore ways to press the heel to the buttocks and catch the foot on your thigh. Explore the access to the hara this catch provides. In continuing out of a catch explore ways you can use that foot to help get you to the other side. Explore all the ways you can follow a catch without losing contact with the foot. Do not combine two kinds of catches. Avoid any torquing of the lower back. If any on the team are comfortable in lotus, explore keeping a foot in your hand as you float their back to your chest and cross their legs into lotus. Explore floating them in lotus. Explore other ways to catch them, such as wrapping them around your waist.

Explore catches in Tandem. While First comes to the feet, Second moves above the head to support. First explores different ways to catch one or both feet against his body as he stretches the legs and/or works with a hip or the lumbar. If lotus or half lotus is comfortable explore crossing the legs and hold him pressed between you. Supine again, open and push apart the legs. Work hara to base.

Round

FIRST FLOATER: Follow Opening and Explore Flow with a catch in which you do one move. Follow the side change with a different catch on the way back to Stillness.
SECOND: Repeat above from side B.
BOTH: Introduce catches in Tandem.

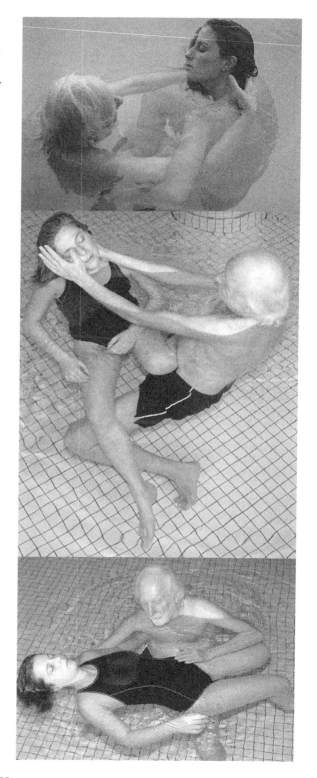

Station 11 Side Tandem

Supporter and Explorer

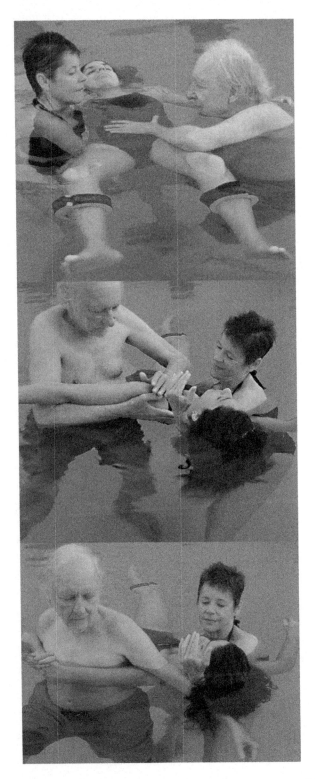

Having concluded each round up to now with exploring one theme from side A while the one at side B supports, those on this path are ready to share the roles in a complete Tandem session. At this station, rather than exploring a single theme, each explores whatever can be done from one side while the other supports. Freed from a Watsuer's constant concern about how the head is being supported, the explorer can engage his whole being in whatever he is holding or moving. The more we engage our whole being, the more the whole being that is reflected in every part of the one we hold is engaged. When we hold an arm or leg to our heart, we are holding more than just the arm or the leg. Explore Wholeness.

The first time you work together with someone follow the progression closely. Later Supporters can add stretches and moves that support whatever the Explorer is doing and roles can be reversed more frequently.

Tandem Side Progression

After the Opening Moves on side A bring the first Explore Flow to a still point

1. The one who had been the witness holds the hara from side B, the right hand below and the left above.

2. Once fully engaged through the breath, the left hand stays and with each inbreath the right hand works up under the back, lifting up into the muscle this side of the spine.

3. When the right hand is under the heart, the left hand joins from above. The two hands hold the heart center between them in stillness for at least three breath.

4. Both hands work the shoulder.

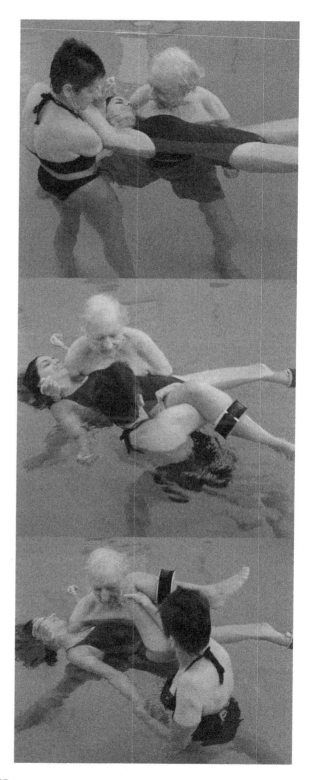

5. Work the arm freely such as reaching over it with both arms, the left working into the trapezius while the right pulls and holds their arm to your heart center.

6. Carry the work with their arm to their leg in a way that maintains continuity such as one hand pushing up under the shoulder while the other pushes the hip (or pulls it reaching around the thigh).

7. Continue exploring rotations and stretches with the leg. In First position invite the one on side A to hold the hara.

8. The one who had been supporting from side A, holds the hara and continues the above progression, 1 to 7, from side A.

Stretching in Watsu

Our goal is not to hold stretches with the intensity and duration required to affect the muscles but to use rotations and stretches to unblock and bring to the surface the flows of energy in our body, and, once it is flowing, to find the stillness within the flow.

Team

With the receiver fully conscious between them, providing feedback, the progression outlined above, skipping the Opening Moves, is done on one side by one and on the other by the other, each exploring in their own way. Each receives once.

Round

FIRST FLOATER: Do the Opening Moves up to Explore Flow and invite second floater to join.

SECOND: Do Side Progression from side B.

FIRST: Do Side Progression from side A.

BOTH: Conclude with Tandem Mirroring led from B and the Tandem Finish.

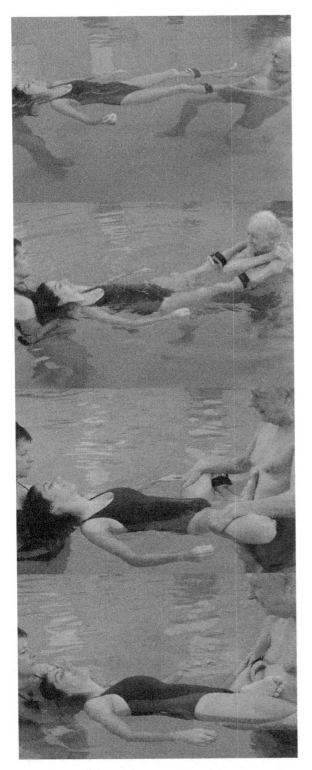

Station 12 Whole Tandem

A Progression in Stages.

In the Whole Tandem on the Explorer Path the progression outlined in the previous station:
Opening Moves, side A
Tandem from the Side, side B, side A
Tandem Mirroring,
is followed by the Tandem from the Feet in which one supports the head while the one who had been on side B starts exploring from the feet. Positioning ourselves between the legs as we stretch them frees the most energy in them. Since the position can be misinterpreted or bring up issues, we approach it in stages that allow us to stay within each person's limits. The Explorer Path Team allows each to discover and express their own limits which are then observed in the Round. Their limits may be respected by not continuing beyond one of four stages

1. Working the feet without opening the legs such as pulling the feet to traction, or pressing the bottoms of the feet to our knees, or holding them to our shoulders to create a wave.

2. Positioning the legs in a way that they remain a barrier to a closer approach such as keeping someone in half lotus while reaching over the legs to work the back, or holding the feet pressed together against our chest.

3. Leaning back against one leg to push out and stretch the other. This is more comfortable for many women than standing between the legs and pushing them apart.

4. Being close enough to the base to reach up with both hands and lift the back, to clasp and rotate the hips and to hold the Hara.

Hara Container

Being close, hands on and under the hara, we contain it from 3 sides. When I first took the stretches of Zen shiatsu into the water the energy they released moved us around the pool. In Tandem that energy is contained, circulating within the one we hold between us. Often when we come to this point and stay, doing nothing, the one holding the hara and the one holding the head (and the one being held) feel that energy moving up the spine.

Waves

Moving the body in waves can start the energy moving up the spine and/or prepare it for a greater move up when someone is held in stillness. In the first stage, if you cross your arms and hold someone's feet to the tops of your shoulders, rhythmically pulling down and back the tops of the feet can start a wave all the way up the back. In the third stage you can rest the knees over your shoulders and start a wave and/or rock them from side to side.

Team

Instead of following the usual rotation in which each is floated once with the others switching roles, each can be floated twice in a cycle that allows them to support and explore before being floated a second time with the roles of supporter and explorer reversed. Explore stage by stage up to whatever limit is found. Explore how the back can be worked, and how the one at the head can explore while the other holds the legs.

Round

FIRST FLOATER: Opening Moves up to Free Arm.
SECOND: Tandem Side from side B.
FIRST: Tandem Side from side A.
BOTH: Tandem Mirroring led from B
SECOND: Tandem from the Feet
BOTH: Tandem Finish.

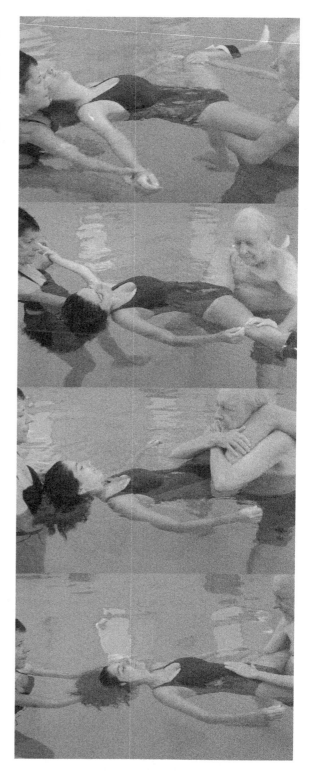

TANDEM WATSU

In 2010 the Tandem Watsu that concludes rounds on the Explorer Path became part of a new Watsu by 3 for couples that combines it with traditional Watsu. Since then Tandem Watsu has evolved into something that, if its intention is made clear, can be offered by itself as a new form of Watsu in spas. Many say that 30 to 40 minutes in the arms of two takes them into a more profound state of being than 60 minutes in the arms of one.

With one person supporting while the other presses and stretches, Tandem Watsu becomes *contained whole body stretching*. Stretching helps unblock the flows of energy through our bodies. Whatever the sources of that blockage, whatever the nature of that energy, most people feel more balanced and a greater sense of peace after stretching.

In acupressure and shiatsu, pressure is applied to points where energy is felt to be blocked. The creator of Zen Shiatsu, Masunaga, says stretching brings that energy to the surface and is a more effective way to unblock and balance it. Watsu began by taking the stretches of Zen Shiatsu into the water. Watsu Free Flow is moving someone through the water to what is felt being released by those stretches.

Because of Tandem Watsu's greater containment whatever is released by its powerful stretches continues to circulate within. The sequence of stretches in Tandem is designed to allow that circulation to continue into deeper and deeper levels, culminating at the moment when, the legs having been thoroughly rotated, opened, twisted and stretched, the watsuers hold in stillness the two ends of the spine, the hara and the head, long enough for whatever is circulating through the body to join whatever might be rising up the spine.

Those who receive a Tandem typically remark at how profound the experience has been. It opens a dimension beyond both bodywork and the traditional ways of working with energy. Watsu's being with someone, not doing something to them, and the safety that containment creates reaches new dimensions in Tandem Watsu's total containment. The energy being released is allowed to circulate within without any attempt to direct it to any part of the body. There is no massaging of any part, no holding of any point to distract or divert its flow. Those being held can apply what circulates through their body to whatever self-healing is needed, or just ride the joy of it.

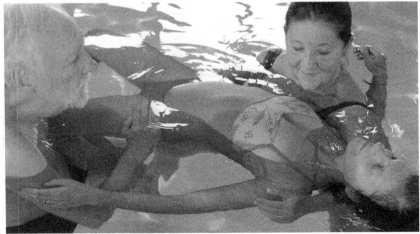

Preparation

Be sure to include among the questions you usually ask someone before a session, questions about their own experience with stretching. Do they do Yoga? Do they like strong stretches? Do they like twists? Have they ever felt discomfort during a twist? Have illustrations of the positions.

Prepare someone who has never received a Tandem Watsu: "This is a new form of Watsu. One of us will start floating and moving you to the breath the way every watsu starts. Then the other will join from the side and stretch your arms and legs every way possible. Because one of us is always here to support the stretches they become very deep, very powerful. Stretching releases blockages. Because of the containment created between us, whatever is released can circulate to wherever it is needed. We avoid any kind of bodywork that might disrupt or distract that circulation. We both remain connected and present, but whatever you feel circulating within is not coming from us. It is a form of your own life force or energy. After the stretches we will stand still, holding at both ends of the spine, doing nothing, allowing whatever has been circulating to join whatever rises up the central channel of the spine, one of us will be holding your head, the other, your hara.

If you feel you would be uncomfortable with one of us between your legs, let us know. we well do all the leg stretches and hold your hara from the side. Also let us know if any of the stretches, or if anything else is uncomfortable. Feel free to let sound or movement from within accompany the stretches. When we finish we will lean you back against the wall. You can stay there as long as you want."

Orchestration

Though the Explorer Path starts out freeing Watsuers from sequence, when two Watsu someone between them they need to understnd how to best exchange and fulfill their separate roles. What follows is a set of steps that help contain what is being released and build up the trust needed to welcome our support at the base. While one maintains support, the other, freed from any attention having to be directed towards keeping the head out of the water, enters into a continuum of holds and stretches in which his whole body is engaged. In the sense that someone's whole body is in every part, when we hold an arm or leg to our heart, we are holding their whole body. This becomes even more of a reality when we no longer have to constantly hold in our attention where the head is. The supporter, freed from having to plan and initiate each move can focus on being present and supporting whatever is happening.

Take your time and work slowly without expectations. Hold stretches until they feel complete. Keep resonance as the base of your presence. If you catch yourself waiting for something while holding the hara do nothing.

Notes

Each column of the following notes describes what one of the watsuers does during a Tandem Watsu. Though any gender could start on either side, to make the notes clearer She is in the left column and He is in the right. One of them is always the supporter (When they are in the role of supporter their instructions are in italics). Side A refers to the left side of the receiver, side B to the right. Receivers are referred to as they. Adapt and develop as needed. The simpler ending below can be replaced by the Tandem Conclusion of the newer Watsu Round.

WATSU BASIC AND EXPLORER PATHS

1	Determine if any conditions call for caution or special attention. Explain process, positions and intention.	
2	**SHE** ... *Stand alongside.*	**HE** ... Say "While she starts, I stay alongside. Let us know if anything is uncomfortable. When movement stops, and you've had time to integrate whatever is happening within, I will join from this side and, working my way around, use my body to hold and brace stretches."
3	Start from side A: Waterbreath Dance, Offerings, Accordion, Spiral Accordion, Free Spine and Gate Hold (clasping the hip gates -the soft tissue adjoining the trochanters- between shoulder and hand) and release into Stillness (arm under, palm down).	*During these opening moves support as a witness from side B. Connecting to the breath, follow, feeling each move in your own body.*
4	When whatever movement Free Spine activated is complete, look up. Silently invite partner to join. *Support in first position, holding receiver close to your heart.*	Approach from side B, moving their arm out of the way if needed. Hold the hara between your two hands, the left on top and the right underneath. When you feel fully connected and ready to explore, your right hand begins gently lifting up under their back. When it is under the upper back, your left hand comes to rest on the heart center
5	*Allow the head to move on your arm in response to his explorations. Avoid any pressure against the neck.*	Hold their shoulder between your hands. Gently lift and roll it, engaging your whole body. Reach over their arm with your left arm. Keep your upper arm pressed against their neck. Hug their arm to you and explore rolls, presses and lifts of arm and hand.
6	Facing right arm, rotate shoulder and hug it close to you. Explore and stretch, as had been done with the other arm. Arrive under the head.	*Support loosely the head in your hand and their body on your arm.*
7	*Hold the head loosely in your hands and support in whatever way allows his moves and stretches to achieve their maximum benefit.*	Reaching over their left thigh and up under the hip, hold the hip gate while your other hand pushes side up toward the armpit. Hold.
8		The thigh still under your left arm, reach down and, holding near the toes, press the heel towards the buttock. Hold.
9		Lifting the leg high, place it over your shoulder. Hug the thigh close and explore moving and rotating the leg.
10	Support head as before until partner has secured the head in his hand. Reach down and, pulling the shin, stretch the bent leg up. Your other hand helps support.	Keeping the leg on your shoulder, work your way far enough up along their side to be able to press the thigh to their chest with your own chest. Holding the press, your left hand reaches over and around the waist. *Your right hand reaches up and holds the head while partner stretches leg up.*

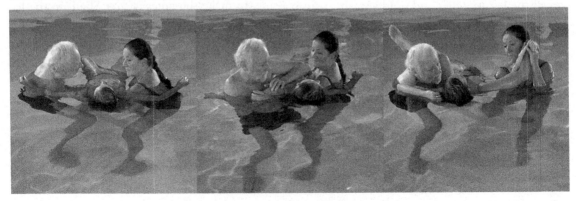

11	*Support head as before.* Pull the bent right leg up to stretch as had been done with the left.	Release the head, gradually unfold the leg, slipping it off your shoulder, and move around their feet to the other side. Repeat the above, 7-10, with their right hip and leg.
12	*Support their head on your left shoulder while your left hand pushes down their left shoulder and your right lifts their right. Gradually increase the twist.*	Lower their right leg and, reaching across, keep their left leg in the water as you bend it up to their side. Swing it up across their body and lean into that bent leg with your left forearm while your right hand reaches under and keeps sacrum pulled towards you. Gradually increase the twist watching their face for any reaction.
	Do not do a twist if anything such as a disc problem counter indicates it.	
12	*Place head on right shoulder and reverse the above to twist to left.*	Straighten the leg, move around to their left side and repeat the above, pulling across and pushing down their bent right leg.
13	*Hold the head without now or later pressing fingers up under the occiput. Throughout avoid any massage strokes or pressure points that might distract or divert the free flow of energy through the body as a whole. Enjoy being there to help contain that flow.*	Hold both ankles and, leaning back, pull the legs straight. Hold. If the receiver has shown any resistance to having the legs open, introduce moves from the left side and explore with both legs held together, now or after 16 below, and hold their hara from the left as when you first joined.
14		Crossing your arms, hold the feet to the outsides of your shoulders and explore ways to simultaneous work the feet and set the body into waves by rocking, pulling the feet.
15	*Continue to support and balance whatever move or stretch is being made.*	Splaying their knees outward, hold their feet, soles pressed together, against your chest. Either reach over and pull their hips towards you, or reach under and pull their sacrum. Hold.
16	Note: This progression is ideal for a Tandem Watsuer to introduce another Watsuer to the support role. If both are experienced Tandem Watsuers they can switch roles as long as one is always supporting. They can explore other moves and stretches as long as they lead up to the hold at the hara that allows whatever is released to work up the spine.	Keeping their right leg folded, its foot resting on top of their left thigh, move up to hold it pressed with your chest while both hands reach under to pull their hips.
17		Releasing the press, back up against their left thigh as your hand or foot pushes and holds out the leg that had been folded.
18		Turning around, fold and press their left leg the way you pressed the right leg.
19		Back up against their right thigh as your hand or foot pushes and holds out their left leg.

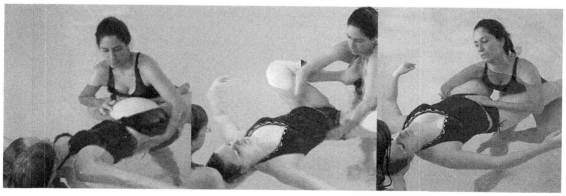

20	~~Hold the head loosely so waves can ascend up through the neck~~	~~Dropping low in the water, slip both knees over your shoulders. Hold~~ the thighs to your chest as you rock back to start waves up the spine. Hold.	
21	*Hold head loosely as it follows the side to side swinging.*	Keeping the knees on your shoulders, stand tall in the water and slowly swing the receiver from side to side.	
22	*If it will improve the support and can be comfortably managed, cross your arms under the head. If you can reach them prop your hands on the shoulder gates (Lung 1).*	Lower yourself back into the water and push out against both thighs. Hold them spread apart.	
23		Move close without pressing against the perineum. Reach up under the back as high as you can, a couple inches to each side of the spine, lift and hold the back up. Lift and hold three or more places working down to the lumbar.	
24	*Hold head loosely in both hands.*	With the heels of your hands press the hip gates from both sides and make small rapid rotations. Come to a sudden stop. Hold the hara, your right hand underneath and your left on top. Stillness.	
25	Explore gentle movements of the head. When that exploration seems complete, catch the supporter's eye.	*Continue supporting with hara between your hands*	
26	Start slowly moving out towards the right wrist without letting go of the head. Hold just below the wrist and pull. (*the Leonardo*)	Move down to the left ankle. Hold and pull.	
27	Changing hands under the head, cross over to the left wrist. Hold just below the wrist and pull.	Cross over to the right ankle. Hold and pull.	
28	Start moving down to side B.	Move up to first position on side A, slipping your forearm under their head, their right arm behind your back.	
	Move into first position on side B, placing your hand under the head just above partner's arm, your other arm below and alongside his right arm.	*Wait*	
29	Hold the receiver close between you and Waterbreath dance together. Three become one.		
30	Close to the wall reach over, hold the thighs, and gently spread the legs to give them a wide base as you lower the feet to the ground. Simultaneously lean the receiver's back against the wall. Place your hand that had been lowering the leg on their chest (Heart Gate). Hold their hand to your heart with your other hand.		
31	Hold the hand that had been on your heart with your middle finger lifting into the center of palm. With your other hand hold your partner's hand likewise, widening the circle. Hold.		

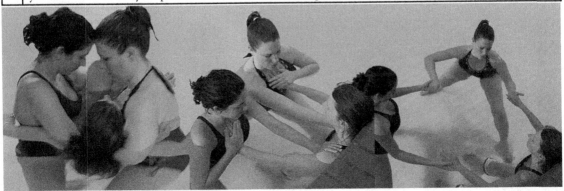

WATSU FOR 2 BY 3 OR MORE

In 2010, watching my students in Goa, my first class in India, seeing how much they enjoyed the short bit of tandem floating that came at the end of each round on the Explorer Path, the idea occurred to me that if a couple were floated by three watsuers, they could alternate between experiencing a regular Watsu, and the new Tandem Watsu, and then at the finish be floated together by all three. I mentioned the idea and before the day was over my students had four couples lined up to come on our last day. I saw each couple having such a powerful experience, I decided to continue exploring this new Watsu for 2 by 3 in my upcoming Watsu 4 in Auroville, a community that, from what I understand, is devoted to union, what better place to explore the power of containment.

By the time I left India eighteen couples had received the new three phase Watsu for Two, including twin sisters and a mother and daughter. Their feedback pointed up the newness/oldness of the dimensions they are taken into both by the Tandem Float and what we came to call the Circle Float in which all the practitioners surround and join them to each other in the last phase. Since we had 15 students in Auroville and a pool just big enough to do three couples at a time, we did all our Watsus for two with five practitioners (two did the first tandem float, another two the second). This can add power to the circle in the third stage but we found that one of the receivers who said she felt ten eyes watching her at the end, might have been more comfortable with fewer practitioners.

Those being floated by two often feel they are being floated by one person, someone that contains them even more than an individual floater could. The more contained they are the deeper they can go within. The more those floating them become one, the more they come to know their own oneness. When the tandem floaters are a man and woman some feel they are being held by their parents. One woman said that feeling her parents become one in the tandem float released her from the pain she had been carrying through the years since they separated from each other. She may have gotten back the support her parents' love for each other had once provided her. The enduring power of love can also appear in an individual watsu. In a recent Watsu a woman who had been quietly sobbing while I floated her explained afterwards that she had got in contact with her love for her father who had died a couple of years before. She was happy to find how much love continues to exist under the sorrow and loss.

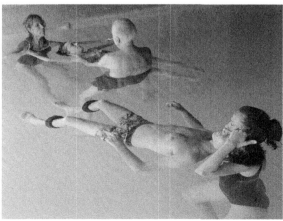
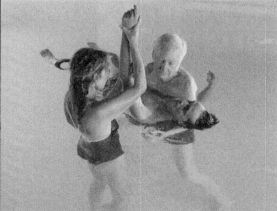

The recovery, the return to a more lasting state of love, often occurs in the Circle Float, where the containment is greatest and the couple can go deep within together. No matter how many practitioners surround and support them they can be perceived as one. One wrote afterwards:

At the beginning I didn't feel I was being floated by one person, as long as I was still aware of the sweet handling of one of them, but very soon it felt like I was moved by an enlarged entity, not very definite but intimate, bringing me through different states. I felt enlarged, projected in a soft deep fluidity, till little by little I started melting, blending with my partner forming a single unit. It was joyous and peaceful

Many said this new Watsu gets them in touch with the essence of their love. This was particularly appreciated by a long term couple who had been having problems for the last six months. Another woman wrote afterwards:

At a certain moment, when they put us together I felt as if I was inside a womb with a twin. I felt such a strong bond with this body that was sharing that reduced space with me, that was affected by my movement as much as I was affected by his movements. Then a very intense emotion came to me and from inside myself there was the need to apologize to my partner for the "shitty" moments that I have given him along the years we have been together. This was followed by a flood of love towards him. It was very intense, very strong.

Another said that the love they felt within the circle would be something that would remain with them to help them through any future difficult moments in their relationship. One man wrote,

Being floated into another dimension, the weight off my shoulders, I remembered the day my mother's heart stopped and my father and I brought her back to life. I felt how much I love my partner and an enormous feeling of safety went through my heart and mind. This experience will always be in my soul and help me through whatever happens in the future.

One couple that had received the Watsu for Two the first time it was offered in Goa and again in Auroville, said that in their first experience they felt their love being restored to the state it had been in when they first met. The second time they both felt and celebrated their connection on a spiritual plane. When a mother and daughter were brought together into the circle of the third stage, the daughter was moved to tears by the love and appreciation she felt for her mother.

When I proposed working with couples in Auroville, some of my advanced students were not

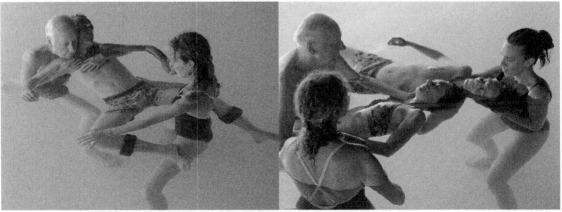

sure they wanted to, but once they experienced this, all recognized its power to unite and move them as much as the couple they held in their circle. One student, after helping hold a couple in a circle in which the love it contained was so tangible it moved everyone, said it was the most powerful experience she had ever had in water. This reiterates what was seen when Watsu was first started, how it affects the giver as well as the receiver, how it gets both in touch with the love that is the foundation of our being.

First Stage: 1 by 1 and 1 by 2

Begin by introducing yourselves and asking each of the pair the same questions a practitioner would ask anyone they are about to watsu. Determine what their previous experience with Watsu, bodywork and stretching has been, and whether they have any problems, including a tendency to motion sickness, that would require attention. Determine if they need float cuffs and, if so, place ones just large enough to keep their knees close to the surface. Explain how after each has received both their tandem float and their individual float, they will gradually be floated closer to each other. When they feel the contact of their partner, they can hold them however they wish or continue to float free alongside them in the Circle Float. Each of the three phases are about twenty minutes. At the end they will be leaned together against the wall.

Have the two stand in the middle of the pool gently leaning back against each other. Tell them to breathe with a single rhythm. The practitioner about to float one individually stands to the right of the one with the least experience of Watsu, a left arm against their occipital ridge. (Whichever practitioner has the least experience with Tandem Watsu will be the one to do both individual sessions.) One of the tandem floaters stands to the right of the other, their left arm against their occipital ridge. On the other side the other tandem floater reaches down and brings the knees of the one they float to the surface in a way that allows both receivers to be gradually lowered into the water into first position.

In the Tandem Watsu follow the same principles and moves described above. Shorten the first floater's opening moves and select the most appropriate from the rest in order to complete the Tandem in its allotted time.

If the individual session is someone's first Watsu, it could begin the same way the practitioner would begin anyone's first. If not, the practitioner could enter into exploration and free flow whenever called to. Balance the more static holding of the tandem float with movement around the pool.

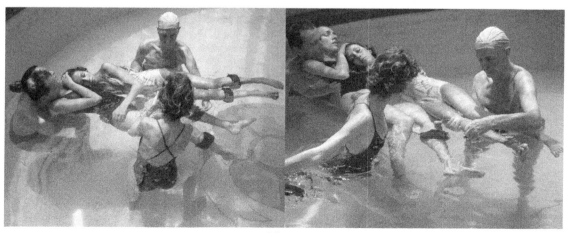

Second Stage: Transfer 1 by 2, 1 by 1

When the twenty minutes of the first stage come to completion:

1. Both those who had started the tandem and individual floats arrive to their receiver's left and hold them out in free float.
2. The one who had joined the first tandem from the left as explorer crosses to the other receiver and enters into first position from the right where he will start as supporter.
3. The individual floater crosses over to the one who had received the tandem float and enters into first position from their right.
4. The one who had been the first tandem supporter crosses over to the other receiver and joins from the left where this time she will start as explorer.

Third Stage: Circle Float

When the twenty minutes of the second stage reaches completion, the practitioners gradually bring the receivers close to each other. Their first contact can be a hand placed in the hand of the other or the tops of their heads touching, or if appropriate, bringing them cheek to cheek. Those containing them arrange beforehand a silent way to move them together. If appropriate, resting the head of one on the heart of the other is a position that lends itself to extended peaceful floating. Bring the one whose head will be on the chest to the left of the other and slip their shoulder under the other's. Take cues from the way they reach out to hold each other to determine how close to bring them together. Hold them floating until the twenty minutes of this stage is complete. Remove any flotation cuffs and keeping them together such as in side saddle or with one leaning against the other who is at the wall. Move to the other side of the pool and wait in your own circle. After they have had enough time to share with each other and look up at you, join and take them standing into your circle where they can share with you whatever they want without any pressure, or remain quiet.

Tandem Watsu From India to Italy

I developed the Tandem Watsu as an offering in itself in the first Watsu 4 after the one in Auroville where I developed the Watsu for 3 by 2. In the meantime, exploring Tandem together with our most experienced Watsu instructor, Minakshi, in the class that she joined and wrote about (page 39), encouraged me to explore further. Another instructor with almost as many years of experience in Watsu, Giordana Valli, invited me to Ischia to give a Watsu 4 to her students. Since all six students worked in spas

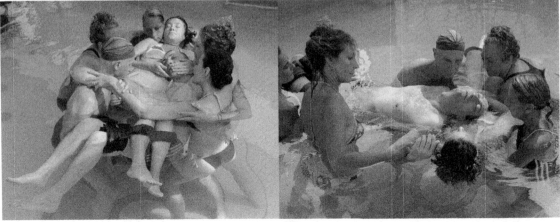

in Tuscany, I started looking at how Tandem Watsu could be offered in spas.

When I first had the students explore the possibilities working in tandem offered, they learned one of its most important principles, that of one person always remaining in a supporter role. I watched a first tandem in which the one who was supposed to remain as supporter started joining the exploration, inventing his own stretches. Seeing their excitement at discovering new ways to stretch someone, I didn't step in. Afterwards the receiver said she didn't enjoy it because all that information coming in confused her body. When the supporter kept to his role of just being there she finally enjoyed being able to completely let go.

In the week that followed, the six with their experience in working with the body and their feedback, helped construct, move by move, stretch by stretch, the ideal order of a Spa tandem. The form that evolved from that first one in Ischia opens this chapter.

The students found a unique value in each of the three of the Tandem Watsu Roles. As the stretcher they could focus on the stretches and their effects as they engaged their whole body without having to be continually conscious of supporting the head. As supporter they could focus on whatever was moving in those they hold without having to keep planning the next move. As receiver they enjoyed and benefited from whatever happened on the deeper level its containment allowed them to enter. Their experience in these three roles helped them reach new levels in the individual Free Flow sessions that remain an important part of Watsu 4.

As Minakshi had done in the earlier class, Giordana encouraged and strongly supported this work. Having practiced and studied yoga and its underlying philosophy in India, and having practiced and taught Watsu for 20 years, she has developed a fine sensitivity to the movements of energy within herself and others. Like Minakshi, Giordana was delighted by the way the Explorer Path takes students and practitioners back to the spirit of early Watsu and wants to become an instructor on that path. As a recipient of Tandem Watsus she felt the canals through which the energy in her own body flows open in ways that were new to her. She feels the role of supporter/witness is as important as its counterpart. As a supporter holding the head, she felt how the energy moved more freely up through those canals when the head was held loosely without the fingertips pulling the occiput. In a Tandem, rather than points, the focus is on the whole body as the embodiment of the whole being and the engagement of our whole body/being in our connection. Giordana introduced me to the Indian

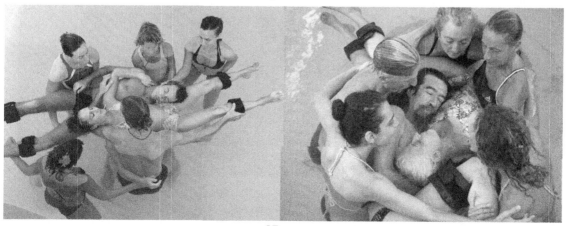

concept of the soft tissue in the hip just beside the greater trochanter, and the corner of the chest at Lung 1, as gates where the spirit enters. Connecting with both has long been a feature in both Watsu and Tantsu. I feel now these Four Gates take on an even bigger role in Tandem Watsu.

The Gates have since taken a central role in this book's Tantsuyoga, the development of which also reached its final form on the same trip to Italy. I feel this new Tandem is too powerful to limit it to those who can afford treatments at spas. Besides continuing to offer it in Watsu 4, I am adding it in a weekend for those who have taken the Watsu Tantsu Explore Flow course.

Finding this most sequenced form of all on a path that started as a path away from sequence may be surprising, but I have experienced, both as a receiver, and as the one supposed to support, how disastrous it is when those working together both go off on their own.

Ireno Guerci, Auroville's official photographer, said he saw more union in our pool than in the hundreds of events and celebrations of union he had photographed.

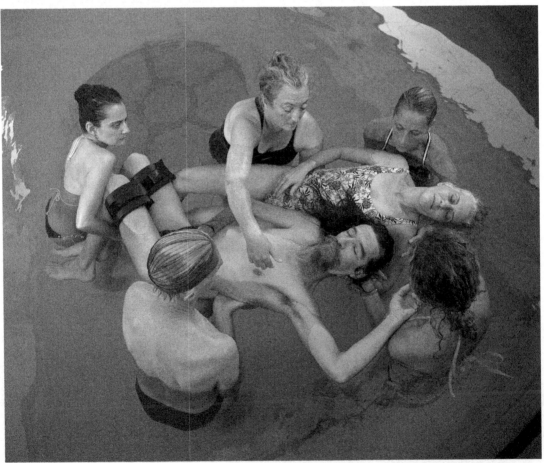

PHOTO: Ireno Guerci

TANTSUYOGA

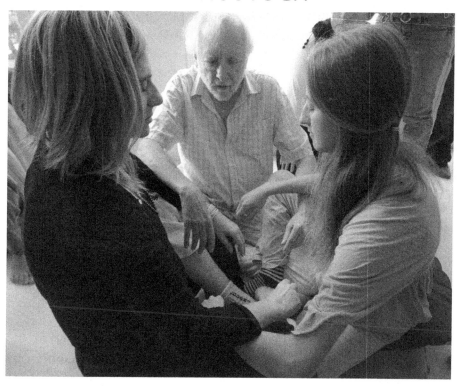

In 2011 I was invited to present at the International Yoga Festival in Milan. To engage as many participants as possible, I developed Tantsuyoga. Three sit with their legs linked, a water flower. Their movement continues beyond the breath, a continuum that draws their linked arms up higher and higher, petals that open as they lean back to the floor. In the round that follows, each has a turn in the three roles, Holder, Held and Helper. With the helper's support the holder can stay longer and keep his eyes closed through the seven celebrations of union. After the festival I introduced this to more than twenty groups in Italy, America and Chile. Everywhere I found people of all ages celebrating the seven levels of union with their eyes closed. Tantsuyoga can be shared anywhere, on the floor or at table. It is one more step toward making the benefits of Watsu accessible to everybody.

Tantsu and Tantsuyoga bring Watsu onto land. In our recent developments of the Watsu Round, the movement as water, continuum, has a greater role. I encourage participants to bring the movement as water into Tantsuyoga.

What follows is a way to introduce this to two others, talking them first through the Round while being in the role of Holder with one, and then with the other. Then join and talk them through the Flower. Follow with the Round again, this time in silence, their eyes closed. If they are new to this, do two turns, taking the role of helper with each. Otherwise start as Helper, and at the end of each of the three turns the helper becomes the next holder. Once all three know this, they can meet again, and enjoy in silence, eyes closed (except the helper) the Flower, the three turns of the Round and the Still Pond in that order.

WATSU BASIC AND EXPLORER PATHS

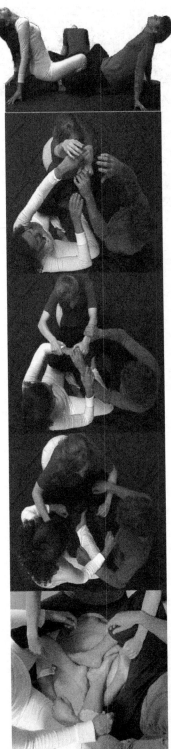

Use the instructions that follow to guide two others from within the Round and the Flower. Start with the Round with yourself as the holder. Describe each of the seven Celebrations. Continue to be Holder in the second turn after Helper and the Held switch roles, speaking again the text if needed. Then, after setting up a massage table if either can't work on the floor, and determining who will receive first in the round (the one who will be on the table if it is set up), join and talk them through the Flower. Then start a new Round as Helper. If they are still learning, continue through two turns as Helper each time, otherwise three turns, silently, with the Holder always being the next Held, and the Held, the Helper. Conclude with the Still Pond.

Water Flower

Have firm cushions in a circle, one for each. Introduce the Flower by saying: "We bring Watsu's engagement with the breath and movement as water onto land. Stand alongside your cushions. Close your eyes. We are standing in water. Hold out your arms. Someone is floating on them. Each time they breathe in they get lighter and draw your breath up, drawing you up through your body center and heart center which become the one core everything is drawn up through. The one on your arms is floating level with your Heart Center. Yoga means union. We are united in the Ocean Within. Rise with that ocean. Open to all sides. Be rooted to the bottom of it, the stalk of a water flower. Be moved to all sides by all the currents around. The Ocean becomes very still.

Open your eyes. Join me sitting in this circle, your left heel in front of your perineum, your right leg over the leg next to you, our feet joined in the center, the root of the flower. Lower your left arm over the thigh straddling your leg. Lower your right arm over the arm resting on your right thigh. Our hands are not touching anything. Close your eyes. Do nothing. We are slowly moved by currents from all sides. We are the fronds of a water plant ... Eyes still closed, take hold of the arm under your right hand. Move it towards the center until our left hands hold each other, the bulb of our water flower, floating on the surface, being moved in wider circles and in and out by the currents ... Water rises ... Slowly lifting us higher and higher... There is nothing left to do but blossom .. Let go with your right hand and reach even higher. THE PETALS OF THE FLOWER OPEN With straight arms drop your hands back to the ground, the front of your body arching up into that celebration... Roll onto your left side."

The Seven Celebrations Tantsuyoga Round

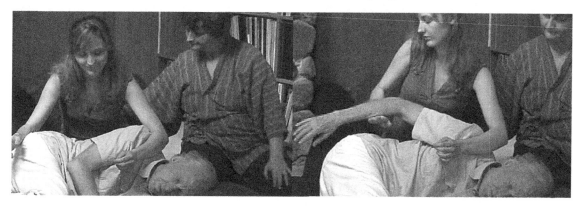

1. Union Within

The receiver is lying in fetal position with her legs as close to her chest as comfortable. The holder sits as close as he can, midway between shoulder and hip, one foot tucked in front, the other leg bent and raised supporting the base of the spine. One forearm in the indentation alongside the trochanter, the other at the softest place at the top of the shoulder, the two arms maintain a gentle constant pressure throughout, allowing them to be pushed apart each time she breathes. The helper places a hand on the holder's lower back where, the holder, eyes closed, says placement and pressure support best.

Yoga means union. In each of our seven holds in this one position, we celebrate an aspect of union. In Watsu when we float someone at our heart our breath is drawn up each time they breathe in and get lighter on our arms. Here, it is when our arms are pushed apart. In both we stay in the emptiness at the bottom of the breath until we are drawn up through our core. Drawn up this way our body and heart centers become one. Their union, the union within, is celebrated in this first hold. Drawn up this way a deeper and longer lasting engagement is established than synchronizing our breathing by watching someone which begins with a separation and ends when we look the other way. Once established, this engagement continues as long as we hold someone.

2. Union Within the Other

The holder reaches out and, without using his hand, lifts the arm and lays it over his right leg. His right arm returns to where it was. His left arm reaches over the shoulder and leans into

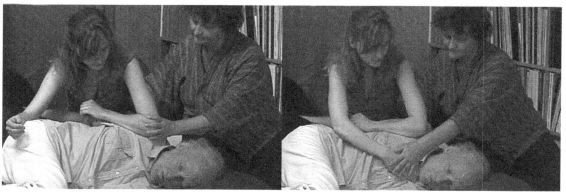

the hollow at the upper corner of the chest.

In India this hollow, and the one alongside the trochanter, are considered gates where the spirit enters. We call them the Heart Gate and the Body Gate. Instead of holding from the outside so that our arms can be pushed apart, in this second hold we are invited into these gates, into the way someone's Body and Heart Centers are continually balancing. In this hold the union within the other is celebrated. Sometimes movement rising within us joins in this celebration. Up to this moment, instead of hands, which have a direct connection to the brain, the holder has used forearms which have an easier time coming from the Core. Now that the Core is engaged the hand can be slowly drawn from the Core to its first place.

3. Union With Another

The holder's hand comes to rest on the Heart Center. His other arm continues to lean into the Heart Gate. That arm is folded the way it is when we hold someone to our heart. Connecting from our Core, with our heart engaged, celebrates our union with another. Instead of movement, in this hold, Union is often celebrated in stillness. Tantsuyoga realizes the basic principle of Zen Shiatsu that Watsu brought into the water, that of being not doing.

4. Wholeness

While the right hand stays stationed on the Heart Center, the other hand, taking the stillness with it, is slowly drawn to the biggest hollow under the occiput, the Mind Gate.

Here, holding body, with our leg still at the base of the spine, and heart and mind, we are holding someone's wholeness, that which is greater than the sum of the parts, with our wholeness. Celebrate wholeness, the union of body, heart and mind.

5. Moving from Wholeness

The Holder firmly clasps the shoulder between both hands and, engaging his whole body, each time he breathes in, moves up and around counter clockwise, a spiraling. The helper, up on one or both knees so that his whole body can join in the movement, places both hands on the holder's back, and, since this rotation is breath timed, breathes with them, as they celebrate moving from wholeness.

6. Ocean

The holder slips his hands, palm up, under the arm, letting the arm lie across his hands, weighing its lightness. Stillness. The holder breathes up his own spine. Without lowering the arm between breaths, the higher the holder breathes up his spine, the higher the arm floats up through an ocean in which we celebrate the ocean within, the whole that is greater than the sum of all the movements within. Each time, the helper's hands are drawn a little higher up the

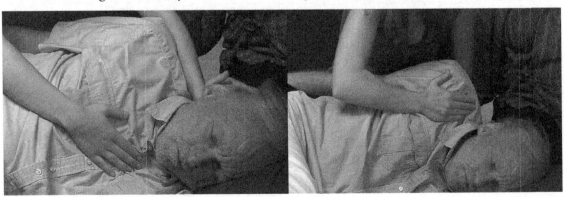

holder's spine. The arm floats up to its highest. The holder slowly moves the arm in all the ways an arm can move in an ocean. The helper moves from his own ocean within. The arm is freed from the ways it is used to control, from its responsibilities, from all it has had to hold onto. The holder appreciates how much is being surrendered, with joy and care, and avoids any bends or twists that would take the arm into an unnatural position and avoids repeated circling or any other movement that is more a doing than a being with.

He lowers the arm up over the head. Avoiding repetitive movement or massage-like strokes his forearms become waves of the ocean rolling their way down the raised arm, finding their way to wherever they are called down the side and the leg and back. The ocean is expansive. Rather than pushing into places they join the ocean's opening. Up on his knees, the Helper's forearms and/or hands accompany with his own oceanic opening on the holder's back.

7. Absence

The holder's hands come to rest just behind the body center and the heart center. The helper's hands come to rest behind the holder's centers. Stillness The helper claps his hands twice; the one held moves just far enough away to be lying in the same position but no longer touched. The helper's hands stay open, no longer touching. The holder's hands stay where they were, no longer touching. Whatever the holder and helper's hands are still holding celebrates the union of absence. The helper claps three times. All three stand and continue as pre-arranged.

Still Pond

After the third turn, all sit again in a circle, legs linked as before, left foot tucked in front and right leg over the leg to the right. This time a cushion is just behind each. Arms straightened behind us on the shore of a still pond, our hands press into the earth's vibrations. Eyes closed, we slowly reach out and press, palm, out, into the stillness over the pond, with one arm and then the other, and slowly cross our arms until our palms meet and press into the palms of those on each side. Hands open, held together by the power of this circle, we are a lotus floating on a still pond. On a still pond there are no currents, no waves to open our petals. It is the light that opens all the flowers, that very slowly draws us up together, that opens our petals.

After blossoming, sit up, eyes still closed, and, move back onto our cushions. Drop back into the emptiness at the bottom of the breath, no longer touching, but still connected. Whatever drew us up out of the emptiness when we held each other continues to draw us up, all the way up into a point of light, light that pours back down into the emptiness.

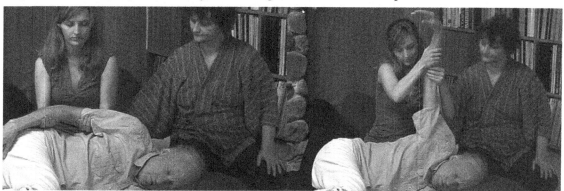

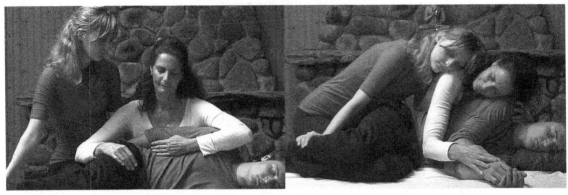

The Posterior Cradle

Holding someone on the floor in the Posterior Cradle can be a challenge for some knees, hips or lower back. Those challenged could hold someone who is lying on a massage table. Minor discomforts on the floor can usually be overcome by the proper use of cushions and repeated practicing. If not, they too could work at a table. Everyone should take responsibility for their own comfort.

To realize the Posterior Cradle's potential for containment, when someone is lying on their left side in as fetal a position as possible, sit midway between their shoulder and hip, as close as you can, your left foot on the floor between you, your right knee raised in a way that helps your leg keep contact with the base of their spine. If the pillow their head is on bulges out behind them in a way that blocks your knee, have them adjust their head's placement, likewise if they have placed a pillow between their knees that blocks the access of your other leg. Maintain contact with the base throughout. If it is broken the one held may feel abandoned.

The kind of cushion you have and how you sit on it can make a difference. If you sit in the middle of a cushion, your back is more likely to collapse. The ideal cushions are zafus, the round firm cushions used for Zen meditation. Sitting on the front edge of them helps you keep the natural curve in your back. Your comfort is also affected by the size of the person you hold. Sometimes a second cushion is needed under the one you sit on. In testing cushions, check them when you have both arms out.

If there is no table available and the traditional Posterior Cradle is uncomfortable try adapting it by bending your left leg back to your left side, or support your left knee on a cushion and keep your left shin under the pillow supporting their head, etc. If no matter how you adapt it there is still discomfort, find someone else to replace your role as holder in the round.

Holding at a Table

Before holding someone at a table, adjust its height for your own comfort. One advantage in working at a table is that you may be able to support their back with your hara. In Tantsuyoga, on the first side, the helper should stand to the holder's right, his left hand on her back while he maintains support at the base of the receiver's spine with either the side of his right forearm, as his hand leans into the table, or his knee lifted up onto the table.

With most people the table works perfectly for the Posterior Cradle in both Tantsuyoga and Core Tantsu. The Anterior Cradle cannot be done at a table, but the Posterior Cradle can be done from both sides. Those working at a table can be in the same round as those on the floor.

Tandem Tantsuyoga

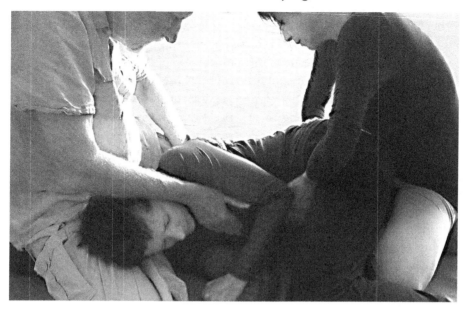

After three join in the Water Flower and all the celebrations up through the ocean on the first side have been done by the holder and helper, continue as follows into a new Seventh Celebration:

7. The Leg

When the holder's right arm or hand has worked its way down the thigh as far as it comfortably can in the Ocean, he looks at the helper. The helper goes to the other side and, up on her knees, takes hold of the foot and knee of the right leg, and keeping it bent, starts lifting it. The holder lowers his right knee to the floor, and slipping his right foot behind him, balances the hip of the leg being handed to him on his right thigh. If the leg's size and flexibility allows it, he holds the leg to his heart center. He moves with it in ways that keep it balanced and grounded over the hip. He keeps himself grounded to the earth. If the leg is flexible enough, the holder can explore stretching it, while the helper holds the knee and foot of the bent other leg. When the holder signals, the helper swings up the bent left leg and leans into both knees, keeping the sacrum flat on the floor while the holder moves above the head, and, makes sure there is a cushion under the head, if needed. He lays the right arm out to the side, and, kneeling, leans into the heart gates. After holding at least four breaths, together, they roll the one held to the second side in a full fetal position.

The Ocean On The Second Side.

The one at the head lifts the head and slips under it in side saddle, his right foot in front and his left to the side. He lays the head on his right thigh while the one at the hip sits side saddle as close as possible, both legs bent, her left foot between them, his upper leg over her left thigh, her right foot out to her side.

8. Holding The Ocean

Once they are settled into their positions, they look into each others eyes and hold out their arms, their right hands, palm down, on each other's left hands, palms up. The movement as water that came in on the first side returns as an ocean they are reaching across, becoming.

9. Hara / Heart

She places her left hand on the hara just below the navel and her right, reaching up behind the back, on a place behind the heart center. He places his right hand on the heart center and his left, reaching down behind the back, on a place behind the hara. They hold, connecting to at least three breaths. The one at the hip always initiates moves. Keeping one hand on hara or heart center, they simultaneously begin a progression with the other hand, he up and she down, the muscle alongside the spine, holding at each outbreath, oceanically moving to the next place during the inbreath, until her hand has found its way into the body gate, his to the shoulder.

10. Hip / Shoulder

Both lay their hands on shoulder and hip and spontaneously synchronize oceanic movement.

11. Down Leg / Arm

While one hand stays in the body gate or the top of the shoulder, the other progresses oceanically with the breath down leg or arm until they simultaneously reach foot or hand.

12. Leg / Arm Up

Reaching under, palms up, they slowly float arm and leg up. Then, holding and flexing foot or hand with one hand while the other hand clasps the knee or elbow, together, they oceanically rotate them.

13. Offering

They offer leg and arm out to each other. Accepting it, they hold with both hands the arm above the wrist or the leg and lean back to pull and hold. They return what was offered and, accepting the return, hook it over their shoulder or hold it to their chest and lean pack to pull and Hold. Clasping the folded leg or arm to their heart center, they join in oceanic movement.

14. Wave

He lays the arm out in front; making sure the one held is fully lateral. She plants the foot on the top of her left thigh or on the floor, and captures the bent knee under her left armpit if possible, or at in such a way that, when she leans back, the back is pulled. Holding it pulled, she reaches behind the sacrum and rhythmically pushes it in a way that sends waves up the back. He has his right hand behind the upper shoulder stabilizing it and the neck, while his other hand, instead of initiating waves, sends those that arrive back.

15. Hara / Heart- Down Leg / Arm

They place hands on Hara and Heart Center and crossing arms behind the back, return to the hold and progressions that opened the ocean on this side, without stopping to rotate shoulder and hip. When they reach the foot and hand, both get up.

16. Completion

Moving above the head, he crosses the arms of the one held and holds the hands to his chest while his other hand makes sure the head is comfortable, slipping a pillow under it if needed. Crossing the arms, he holds them below the wrists while she takes hold of the heels. Both squat back to pull. She lowers the heels to the floor and leans into the tops of the feet. He holds the occiput and pulls. She holds the feet turned out to the sides, the heels of her hands in the soles. He lightly rests his palms over the eyes without touching them, blocking out all external light. He lightly lays his hands on the heart center and the third eye. They simultaneously lift their hands off. They continue sitting, focusing on how the three are still connected though no longer touching. They may choose to join in the StillPond.

Recognizing the benefits that come from

Tantsuyoga Presenterships

unconditional holding and the need for it around the world, a YouTube and directions for any three to join in a Flower Round are posted at www.tantsuyoga.com, as well as directions for leading groups of any size through it.

Typically there are two parts to a presentation to a group. In the first hour the round with its seven celebrations is demonstrated describing the union being celebrated in each. Then participants take turns in the roles, each being quickly chimed through the seven celebrations with their eyes open. At each turn of the round, help is provided the holder to find the most comfortable way to hold someone on the floor or at a table,

Then, with new partners, they are slowly chimed through the seven with their eyes closed.

In the second hour, the moves of the Water Flower are demonstrated. All stand, move as water. Then, sitting, linking legs and arms, all join in a single Water Flower. When its petals open, participants continue in the round in silence as they are chimed through the seven celebrations, eyes closed. All link legs as in the Water Flower, but this time reaching across a Still Pond. When the petals open, no longer touching, they sit in a circle and follow whatever drew them up out of the emptiness when they held someone, all the way up to a point of light, light that pours back down into the emptiness.

If Presenters regularly offer this, participants can be invited to return for just the silent second hour. Directions for Registering their Presentership will become available at tantsuyoga.com.

If there is a pair registered to offer Tantsuyoga for Two and/or a Tantsu practitioner, contributions and income they generate could help support the regular offerings of the Flower Rounds to the public which in turn will draw clients to the sessions.

Help realize our goal of making unconditional holding and the ocean within accessible to everybody.

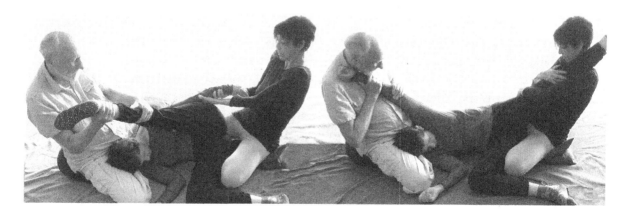

TANTSU

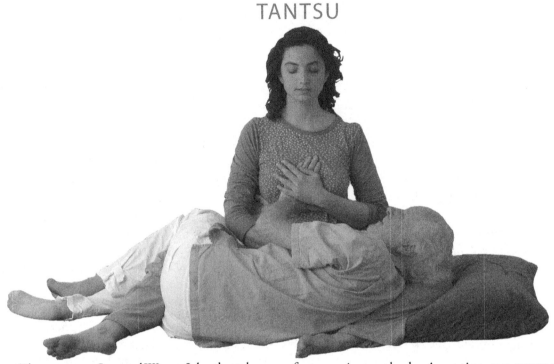

The same year I started Watsu, I developed Tantsu to bring Watsu's unconditional whole body holding back onto land. I was teaching Zen Shiatsu and developed Tantsu moves that could be combined with it or joined together in a complete Tantsu. In Zen Shiatsu we use our weight as we lean in. In Watsu we are under someone holding them. In Tantsu our leg supports someone's base throughout most of its cradles and stretches, adding to the containment within which those held feel safe.

Containment is the oldest form of healing. It brings peace to the fallen infant picked up and held to his mother's heart. Those who experience that peace in Tantsu often comment on how safe they felt, and how that containment allowed them to go deeper within. Our calf is ideal for maintaining the support at the base. Its role in our own life is to support us. It is far from our mind and its intentions.

The base is at the source of many of the flows of energy in our body. Accepting our support there may help some accept their body as a whole with its place in the union of their whole being. Some who have had the support at the base inadvertently removed during a Tantsu, even if it is only a few inches of separation, have commented on how they felt abandoned. It may be that the constancy of this support is at the base of the peace we find in Tantsu.

Illustrated above is Tantsu's first and most powerful position, the Pieta. In a complete Tantsu it usually comes at the end of the session after many holds and stretches.

In 2006 I was invited to Chicago to teach Tantsu to a group of Tantra teachers who had read my first book, Bodywork Tantra. When they told me of the success they had helping couples who learned to hold each other with just the Pieta, I decided to develop a new form of Tantsu for people that were already close enough to start with the Pieta.

With the help of one of the Chicago teachers, Amber Seitz, we held Tantsu classes with just the Pieta in America, Switzerland, Italy, Spain, France, and Holland. Everywhere we found that even those who were not intimates were comfortable in the Pieta. Though most feel safe once they are in the Pieta, not everybody is comfortable starting in it. I developed the Posterior Cradle to contain and work one whole side from the back, and build up trust, before rolling someone into the Pieta (Anterior Cradle) to work their second side. I was surprised to find the way our arms are pushed apart each time someone we hold in this new cradle breathes, draws our breath up, draws us up out of the emptiness. It is the Waterbreath Dance on land. It unites body and heart centers as one core. I call it Core Tantsu.

In 2008 an Italian publisher asked me for a Tantsu book. **Tantsu,** *A Yoga of the Heart*, features both the new Core Tantsu that anyone can share, and all the cradles that can be included in a complete Tantsu or a Zen Shiatsu session. While teaching Core Tantsu in India I was told that Yoga means union. I realized that, instead of being a bodywork that separates giver and receiver, or isolates parts of the body to be fixed, this is a whole-body bodywork that celebrates union.

When I first heard the concept of oneness, that we are all one, I scorned it. As a young poet and a budding connoisseur of the arts I was drawn to the uniqueness of each event or person. Then in Zen Shiatsu I learned to lean into two places and drop into the emptiness at the bottom of the breath where they become one. I learned to feel the energy released when we stretch someone. I took those stretches into the water and felt oneness with whomever I floated at my heart, and whatever the stretches released drew me around the pool in Free Flow.

A year or two later, I slowed down to enjoy the newly discovered emptiness at the bottom of the breath in the Water Breath Dance. We find our deepest peace in that emptiness. The more the breathing of the one in our arms draws us up out of it, the more the centers we are drawn up through become one, the more we know our wholeness, the more the one in our arms knows their wholeness, a knowledge we are kept from by whatever imbalances we are subject to. Many therapies focus on the imbalances, whereas the paths in this book start with the wholeness of both the holder and the held.

I find the wave drawing us up strongest when we sit in a circle that Watsu or Tantsu has bonded into a wholeness, and I lead us up into a point of light. When all that light pours back down into the emptiness, the wave bounces me off the floor. The wave is not a release of tension but the ground of our being. Like the particle and wave in physics, emptiness and the wave are two states of the same event, our wholeness.

Posterior Cradle

Have someone lie on their left side. Position yourself behind them as in Tantsuyoga and go through the first six celebrations. Since there is no one supporting your back, let yourself move whenever you feel the need. Wherever the forearms and/or the hands establish themselves in Tantsuyoga, after connecting through the breath in stillness and letting your body move from within, explore how either one of your arms or hands remain as a station while the other is drawn wherever called. After working down the back and leg, stand, and, without straining, swing both knees up. Lean into the knees, keeping the sacrum flat on the floor. Roll them to their right side and, having prepared them beforehand to help if needed, position their head on your supported left thigh and bring your right leg around their pelvis.

CHECK Make sure they are lateral without their right arm pinned, that your leg under their head is fully supported, as are you, raised high enough to reach around them, and another cushion is behind them to later support their arm. Having told them beforehand to make whatever adjustments are needed to stay comfortable once they are in the Anterior Cradle, encourage them to adjust as needed now or anytime later.

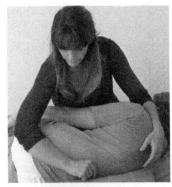

FOREARMS Once you and your partner are well established, without strain lean forward and rest your forearms on the least bony places you can find on the side of the hip and the top of the shoulder. Without applying pressure nor holding, your hands continue to hang limp behind your partner. Drop into the void at the bottom of the breath. Wait for their in breath to push apart your arms and draw you up out of that emptiness. Breathing in, notice whatever tendency to move rises up and out into your arms around them. If there is movement let it unfold in whatever way it wants. If not, continue enjoying holding in the stillness.

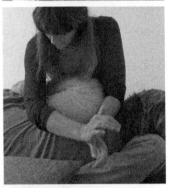

SHOULDER Keep one forearm at the top of the shoulder. Place the other against the shoulder and lift and roll the shoulder. Explore, moving from your core. Replace your forearms with your hands one at a time. Without stopping the movement push the shoulder so that their arm slips behind their back and rests on the cushion behind them.

PUSH PULL Your left hand pushes against the top corner of their chest (not their shoulder) while your right hand reaches over and gently pulls the muscle in the lower back (unless a disc problem countraindicates this gentle twist). Hold at least three breaths.

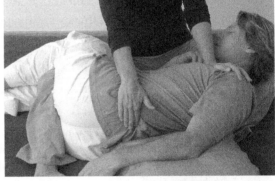

ROCK BACK Both hands reach over the back, side by side, as high up on the back as they comfortably can without putting pressure on the arm they are reaching under. Fingertips are close to, but not touching, the spine. Hold. On an outbreath rock back, your arms straight, pulling your partner's back as you lean way back releasing your own back. On the inbreath rock forward and, keeping your left hand where it is, place your right hand three or four inches further down the back. On the outbreath rock back again. Repeat slowly rocking forward and way back until your hand reaches the sacrum Return your lower hand to its place alongside the upper hand.

EXPLORE DOWN BACK Keep your left hand at its station in the upper back while your right hand explores down alongside the spine moving with whatever motion, pressure and pace that feels inviting.

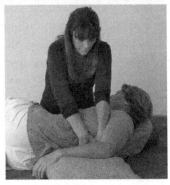

CORE TANTSU ANTERIOR CRADLE

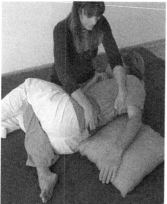

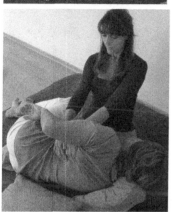

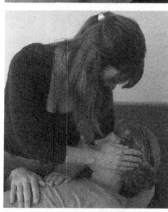

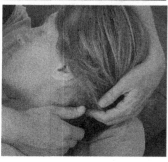

SPIRAL As you breath in pull the upper back towards you with the hand closest to the head. As you breathe out pull with the hand that starts alongside it. Continue pulling with the hand closest to the head on each inbreath and with the other, moved a little further down the back, on each outbreath. As you alternately pull with each arm feel your body engaged in the pull by a spiraling up into your shoulders. When the descending hand reaches the sacrum, maintain its hold on the lower back while your left hand, reaching between your waist and their face, arrives at the heart station. Hold.

The above are three different ways to release someone's back. Keep your left hand at the same station during all three phases. Feel free to explore down the back with any of them more than once, in which case the rhythm could become more dynamic and build up.

HEART STATION Your right hand continues its gentle and steady pull of the lumbar. Your left stays on the heart center. Hold. Be aware of containing and breathing with their whole body. Keep that awareness in your right hand. Release its pull. Coming from your core, it gradually approaches their face and comes to lightly rest on their cheek. Hold.

AROUND THE HEAD Keep one hand on their heart as the other gradually works its way up and around the face and the head. Wherever you touch or hold or move it is not just that place you touch but their wholeness. And you are touching with your core. Each time you feel completion in your core let yourself be drawn to the next place.

OCCIPUT When your right hand arrives at the occiput, lift your left hand up and over their head to hook their occipital ridge. Pull the ridge, while your right hand presses the muscles down the side of the neck, works under the scapula and pulls the top of the shoulder. Hold.

ARM BREATH SQUEEZE Lay their arm on their side, Hold the top with your left hand while, leaning in further down the arm with each outbreath, your right hand presses and squeezes the breath out of the arm (and your core). Just before it reaches the wrist, after you lean in on the outbreath pick up the arm as you breathe in.

FREE EXPLORATION Let the arm lie across your open hands. Find a point of balance. Listen. Move, stretch and hold in whatever way invited. If you lay it stretched up over the head, explore spreading their side with crossed arms and the access into the lower back provided. Explore what can be accessed in each position. Explore hooking your fingers under the scapula or along the spine as you lean back. When complete hold the hand in both hands. Contain and explore.

HEART HEART Hold their hand, palm towards you, to your heart center with your right hand while your other hand rests on their heart center, having arrived there with your arm between their head and your waist. Hold. Feel how deeply connected your cores are. Hold

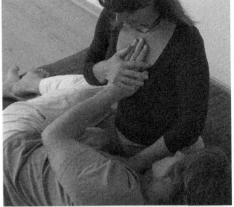

HEART HARA Keep your left hand on their heart. With your right hand either lay their left arm over your right thigh or behind their back (supported on a pillow if needed). If their other arm is blocking your way to their hara, move its forearm toward their chest. Place your right hand just below the navel, pushing in with more pressure than the constant pressure the left hand maintains at its station at the heart. Keeping your back straight, hold both until they too become one at the bottom of the breath.

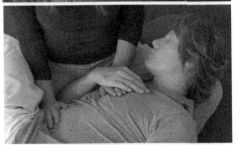

HARA HARA Remove your left hand from the heart and, reaching over their back, pull their lumbar towards your right hand which is still pressing from the front. Notice how, with your right leg's continuing support, you are now holding the base of their core from three sides. Hold their whole core as one.

HIP When that feels complete, keep holding the back of the Hara with your left hand while your right hand reaches over to come to rest alongside it. Hold. Keeping your left hand at its station, explore movement around the hip. Explore with both hands. Rock back pulling the hip. Move and rotate the hip gradually increasing the speed. With the heel of your right hand press into that softer indentation where you first rested your forearm and vibrate.

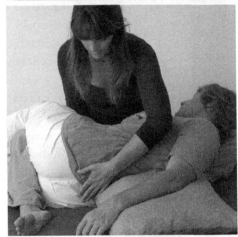

DOWN LEG Place your left hand just below your right and explore down side of leg with right hand or forearm pressing gently with each outbreath into a new place without sliding.

FREE EXPLORATION Pick up and hold the leg by the foot and knee. Find and maintain its balance as you explore rotations, lifts. stretches, and whatever invites as you clasp the leg to your chest or hook it over your shoulder or prop it.

BACK BEND If flexible enough, bring their left foot behind them and hook it back with your right foot to hold the stretch. Hold the lumbar with your left hand as your right gently presses down the front of the thigh. With this stretch maintained their body itself becomes a station, a station you can explore gently pulling with your hands up and down their back.

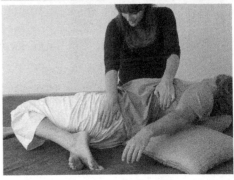

CORE TANTSU ANTERIOR CRADLE

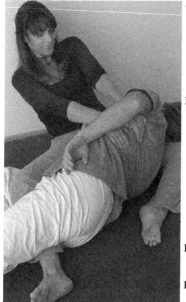

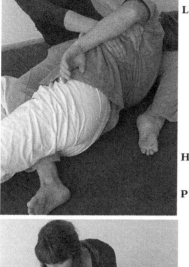

THREE PHASE ROCK DOWN TO LEG After straightening the leg from the back bend, anchor one hand in the upper back and rock as in the Rock Back, Explore Down Back and Spiral, continuing each phase as far down the hip and leg as you can comfortably reach. As you complete the third phase, continue into the Leg Roll

LEG ROLL Hold the lower back with your left hand while your right hand without gripping pushes and pulls the top of the leg, getting the leg to roll on its own as much as possible. When the right hand has gradually worked its way down to the knee, the left is lightly placed on the hara just below the navel while the right slowly works its way back up pushing against the inner side of the thigh. When it is almost at the top of the leg, it crosses over the other hand to come to rest on the Heart Center.

HARA HEART With arms crossed hold Hara and Heart. Drop into stillness in your own Hara. Hold.

PULL UP ARMS Lift up near arm and hold it to your heart as you lean back. If your leg is trapped under their thigh, slip it out free while keeping your shin's support at their base. Lift up the far arm and hold both arms with your right hand, pulling them enough to slip your leg out from under their head which your left hand gradually lowers to the floor. Lower their arms as you slip back, disengaging.

FINISH Straddle and press both knees towards chest keeping sacrum flat on floor. Lift legs and, holding by the heels, squat back to pull. Lower feet and press down just up from the toes. Hold. Lean both hands into insteps pressing feet outwards. Hold. Leaning in, work up legs to Hara and, without losing contact, pick up left arm. Walk around their head and pick up right arm. Squat back to pull crossed arms. Pull occiput. Cover eyes. Hold heart and third eye. Lift up both hands. Sit. Meditate on how you are still connected without touching.

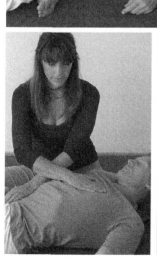
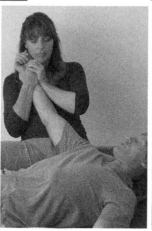
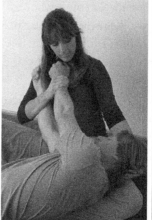
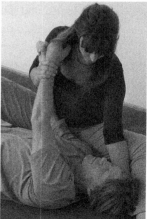

ON THE PATH

I watched a lecture in which Jill Bolte Taylor explained the separate functions of our brain's two hemispheres in a way that rounded out my understanding of Watsu and our path. She is a Harvard brain scientist who had a stroke that gradually disabled the left hemisphere. With the right hemisphere still functioning she experienced a state of being that was totally in the moment, being one with the energy of the universe with no sense of boundary. It took several years to relearn language and the full functioning of her left hemisphere. She explained the right hemisphere engages in our immediate sensations which being completely in the moment have no limit. The left is linear and, able to compare current sensations to past, builds language and our identity, reasons and plans futures.

I see these as two minds, our being mind and our sequential mind, that, throughout our lives integrate with varying degrees of success with our other two, our heart mind (our connecting mind) and our body mind (our survival mind). Each of the four, can become dominant in our lives.

Reasoning may dominate at times, but when the sequential mind becomes most dominant is when an irrational idea, or an obsession, or blind faith in a doctrine engages it in continually adjusting reality to support that belief.

The Being mind can dominate in those who leave the world behind to devote themselves to a practice that shuts off the chatter of their left brain.

The Heart mind, with its own neurons and brain, takes over when we fall madly in love. It is engaged in our emotions with those we connect to. With no one to connect to the heart is at risk.

While continuing to maintain our breathing and circulation in the background with the autonomic nervous system, our Body mind can become dominant in many ways. Its oldest strategy for survival, reproduction, can turn our lives around. At other times it can become obsessed with the preservation or performance of our body in athletics, fitness, dance or yoga. It may also be involved when we are unable to decide between what the heart and our rational mind want and get our answer through a gut feeling.

All four of these minds are engaged in both giving and receiving a Watsu. The way that engagement comes into place may help characterize and distinguish the different forms of Aquatic Bodywork. I still remember my first experience with being taken underwater in Waterdance and my fear the student practicing it on me wouldn't bring me up to breathe when I needed. Then I received a session from Waterdance's co-creator Arjana, which took me so far beyond that fear I forgot any need to breathe. I felt completely one with the water. There is a moment when we start a Watsu, when we sink up to our chin and wait so deep in the bottom of the breath, that we forget we are waiting for the breath to draw us up. Both are moments in the Being mind. In my own experience giving Waterdance I found myself having to stand higher out of the water to guide and stay attentive to the needs of the one under. In Watsu it is the giver who drops deepest into the water and lets it do everything. It is beginning at that depth in the Being mind that characterizes Watsu and establishes it as a path for the giver.

Watsu begins in the emptiness at the bottom of our breath. The coordination of the movement that follows to our shared breathing helps someone surrender control and access their own Being mind. The movement that comes out of emptiness leads to a stillness in which our Heart minds connect as the movement within joins in the flow. Our Being, Sequential, Heart and Body minds are all engaged on this path. The more integrated they are into the flow, the more likely they are to reach greater integration in both of us. To the degree that, as in any form of art, the whole is greater than the sum of its parts, their integration can engage a fifth mind, our Wholeness mind. When I stand in front of a masterpiece it is not the beauty of what is depicted but the wholeness the painting emanates that brings the greatest joy to my own wholeness mind. Wholeness is the path and the vehicle of integration that carries us on it is the creative.

Other Paths that led to the Watsu Path

The paths that I look back down arrived at a greater wholeness when the sequential mind surrendered its tendency to dominate. The first path that I recognized as My Path was poetry. On graduation I joined the poets flocking to San Francisco. When I read him the poems I had written at the university, Jack Spicer said they sounded like I had the last line in mind when I started writing them. It was true. My sequential mind had been well trained in academia. Stepping beyond it, words and images come with a spontaneity that creates a new level of connection.

A 'last line' can get in the way on another path that winds in and out of our lives, a path that sometimes has more to do with the body, and sometimes the heart. If, while making love, we connect to, lock into, the energy rising in our partner, we can go beyond that need for a 'last line' as heart and body reach a new level of integration.

Connecting to the energy in another while leaning into and stretching them in Zen Shiatsu opened still another path, a path that led into the water.

One night I was floating someone in the warm pool. Then she floated me. As I lay on my back waves started vibrating my whole body. When I stood up I felt a rising all the way up into a world of light. I wanted to take others to that place. I floated others. In Zen Shiatsu I had learned how stretching can bring energy to the surface. As I stretched those I floated, I followed each stretch with the movement I felt the energy released by the stretch led me into. There was no sequence. Occasionally those I floated would have the kind of wave in their body that had started me down this path. The wave in my body would resonate to theirs. At the end when I lifted both hands up off their third eye and crown chakra, we rose, two dragons intertwining together up into the light.

There were always people willing and eager to be floated and stretched in that warm pool. I did find myself being drawn to women, but whether I floated women or men I realized the connection and the energy being shared has nothing to do with gender. This was the heyday of the sexual revolution, at a hot springs near San Francisco where clothing was optional. Being so readily available, sex, or rather the seeking of it, did not get in our way of just being with someone, particularly when we had so much trust placed in our arms. Someone floating in them, naked and surrendered, can be very beautiful and, as with a work of art or a poem, it is their wholeness that is the most beautiful, what can not be violated.

The safety felt in those first Watsus helped establish the closeness and whole body holding that characterizes Watsu. The closeness made it possible for our body to brace Watsu's most powerful stretches. Flotation devices had not yet been developed, and the more someone tended to sink, the more we had to stay low in the water and use our whole body to help support them. As Watsu evolved its closeness helped us connect moves to the breath and access the movement within. Besides continuing to support stretches, its whole body holding helped us develop rolls and other powerful moves.

I started showing my Zen Shiatsu students how to float and stretch each other. I tried to show them all the different ways to stretch someone that I had been discovering, but the more I showed them, the more stressed they became feeling they had to learn, to memorize all of them. To help them I developed a sequence. In Zen Shiatsu we connect to someone's breath, leaning into them as they breathe out, something we can't do in the water. I developed the Water Breath Dance in which we connect to someone's breath as they breathe in. It was waiting to be drawn up out of the emptiness in the bottom of the breath where Watsu truly began. Having students start in their Being mind as a wide range of moves connected to the breath evolved while their feet stayed grounded in the same place helped them to be present. But staying present as their Sequential mind focused on learning a sequence was difficult for many, particularly with the first sequence where I tried to put every move into one week. I extended it over two weeks… and then three.

Learning from the Sequence

In learning a form there is a stage when it is no longer just the sequential mind that is engaged. When the body mind has learned the form more of our being can become engaged as the moves unfold without having to plan them ahead. We no longer have to think about what comes next. We become more attentive, more responsive, to how each move is applied, and adapted to the one in our arms. Many feel challenged at first learning the Transition Flow of Watsu 1. The moves in a transition that takes you from one position to another need to be followed in the order that insures you get where you want to. Once your body has incorporated the transitions everything flows into place and you can explore what you can or cannot do in each of these positions. Having divided the instruction into three separate weeks in which a complete form, and how to adapt it, has been learned by the end of the second week, leads some students into confusing Watsu with that form. Watsu is not the sequence.

In the third stage, Watsu 3, the form is left behind, but not what it has taught your body about being with someone in the water. The more your body has learned, the freer it is to enter into Free Flow with someone, the more likely your body is to be where it is needed when someone you lift into the air in one of the rolls of Watsu 3 rolls back down, the more likely it is to take someone off into completely new directions. The more your whole body is surrendered into Free Flow the more their whole body becomes engaged and spontaneously calls you to places or moves or new rhythms or stillness.

The body being freed in the subtitle to the book Watsu 'Freeing the Body in Water' is as much that of the giver as the receiver. The engagement of both was even more explicit in the title of my first book to introduce Watsu and Tantsu, 'Bodywork Tantra'. I have since left Tantra out of the title to avoid denying Watsu's benefits to those who confuse Tantra as a form of sex. Sex is just one of the many arts into which Tantra can come into play. Tantra is the creative engagement of our life force. There are many paths.

Learning from the Flow

From the time we introduced the Waterbreath Dance, I felt the difference between what rises up out of the emptiness at the bottom of the breath from what moves through someone's spine when we hold them out in front of us in what we now call Distant Stillness. Both are clearly different from the movement that comes through our heart and out are arms from our whole core when we hold someone close, what we call Explore Flow. In the past, as described above, this was not introduced, or rather not focused on, until the student had fully incorporated the sequence into their body and came to Watsu 3.

Just as introducing the Water Breath Dance slowed students down enough to connect their breath to what lifts whoever they hold and continue that connection into movement, Explore Flow leads to a continuum of movement that engages the whole being of both. Now, by having students experience and explore both breath timed moves and Explore Flow in Basic Watsu before they have to learn any sequence, can start them learning from their wholeness mind and create a presence that will stay with them as they incorporate the steps of a sequence.

Empty, explore, encounter, engage. The exploration continues into a flow in which we encounter the spontaneous, a move from nowhere, or a call to someplace on the one we float. The more we surrender into those moves and answer those calls with our whole being, the more our whole being becomes engaged. With someone in our arms, the spiraling path of our creativity becomes a double helix that engages the whole being of both.

Sharing all these various flows of our life force, as well as those released in powerful stretches and waves, frees us from any temptation to fit them all into a single theory. To the degree that encountering, experiencing deeply in our own being, what can not be explained frees us from seeking, or accepting, anything that pretends to explain everything, this is a path of freedom.

Usually those who start out on a path have a goal in mind. Explorers setting out from the old world to the new sought gold or the fountain of eternal life. On this path there is no last line. If our Sequential mind can surrender its need for one, it can integrate with our Being, Heart and Body mind on the path that is our wholeness, and we can, for a moment, share our birthright in the creative vibrancy of this universe.

The Path Back

I have been enjoying the longest season in my home over the stream since I started traveling around the world to teach Watsu. It has been a time to go back to sources, the Greek world of Homer, Herodotus and Socrates on one hand, and the painfully wrought poetry of Jack Spicer on the other. No matter how deeply I ensconce myself under these lush woods my stream feeds, when reading and writing wanes, the internet reconnects me to today's world, both in my work with the Water Family, and its daily reporting of everything that is happening.

When the internet first came into our lives I welcomed it as a powerful tool of education, but as Socrates shows, education is learning to ask questions. Instead of questions the internet pumps out the fly by night merchants' answers to all our physical conditions, the shock jocks' answers to all our social ills, and the fundamentalists of each religion's answer to everything.

The world's first democracy had its answer to all of Socrates's questions, the poison in the cup they forced him to drink. But that was no more an answer than what Jack Spicer drank himself to death with. There are no answers. Whatever we believe we believe is open to question. There is only the flow. Every time I look out my window I am looking at a new stream.

The question remains: what underlies the need to have something that answers everything? Is it fear, and if we have the four minds proposed above, does the same fear interfere in their integrating? Does each of the four have its own fear to isolate it? The Sequential mind- the fear of losing control? The Heart mind- the fear of abandonment? The Body mind- the fear of physical decay? The Being mind- a fear as deep as that of falling? And when there is wholeness, are all those fears contained within it? Or are they patiently waiting outside? And does the knowing how momentary our wholeness must be make it all the more precious, all the more beautiful to share with others on this path?

CONTRIBUTIONS BY FABRIZIO AND ATEEKA

Fabrizio Dalle Piane brought years of experience with, watsu, continuum and other movement arts to help develop core tantsu and the watsu explorer path. Ateeka, an artist and Yoga instructor, brings her background with continuum and her experience in creating a yoga that incorporates flow. She has developed a Somatics Educator training that features a Tantsu that incorporates the internal dimension presented here.

THE ART OF THE SOMATIC DIALOGUE

How "Explore Flow" differs from "Free Flow"

A Watsu Explore Flow session is a "multi-lingual" endeavor, in which our range of communication may extend from spoken sharing to subtle perception of the silent inner flow. While the practice is without goal, in order to deepen into the two-way communication, we can engage in a "dialogue" rather than monologue with our partner(s). The "somatic dialogue" is an ongoing exchange of information between the practitioners' inner movements and the outer explorations that manifest. The communication of this "somatic dialogue" is wide and vast and has the potential to go beyond the "role" of personal identity. It is truly the language of the body and the heart.

The language of the body is both primordial and cosmic. It is ancient and it is future. It lands us in the "right-here-and-now." In order to communicate deeply with our partner(s) in an Explore Flow session, we need to become fluent in the language of the body.

The language of the heart is one of coherence. It is when we are able to let go of our ideas of right and wrong and melt into the feeling sense of truly being with another. It is empathetic. It is our first language. We cannot "learn" this language of the heart, as it is already within us, we simply can re-member its soft, natural and very healing tone. The simple act of being with another in a Watsu exchange can help us to access this universal language.

Traditionally, when learning a language, we go to a school or out on the streets of a new country and seek to "acquire" new words, phrases or pronunciations. In learning the language of the body and the heart, the most important step is learning how to perceive and receive. We slow down and first listen to our own inner presence. The first step is a bit like this: imagine yourself walking in a thick overgrown forest, immersed in all of its activity, and as happens, it suddenly occurs to you that you have lost your way. With no compass in your pocket, you must tap your natural instinct in order to find your way. You stop where you are, take a breath, get silent, listen and follow your way to the sound of running water, which is a flow that will give you a direction to follow and keep you from "walking in circles"

The spirit and source of Watsu Explore Flow is much like this. The "direction" we follow originates from the inner (often fluid) movement of who we are holding. We slow down, breath, get still, listen and shed expectations to really sense our partner in all of his/her humanness. It is only then that we can truly "follow movement". The uninterrupted following movement is born of the resonance of the two or three people engaged in the sharing. Follow Movement is a "somatic dialogue" of non-doing in the presence of the not-knowing. Talk about limitless possibilities!

"Follow movement" often grows into "explore movement". This phase in the Watsu Explore Flow cycle is not just "exploring some new moves" that an outside source (teacher, book, video, other) has suggested. It is the authentic engagement of our shared life force energy in a playful and curious way. It is respectful, joyful, surprising and neurologically enriching. Explore Flow is different from Free Flow. True Free Flow originates from being highly skilled and practiced the various moves, holds, techniques of Watsu and being able to use them in spontaneous and highly creative ways.

Explore Flow comes from within. It is born of the moment. It is always innovative and its source is not dependant on one's skills, experience or level of practice. Of course, some basic foundation skills of how to hold and simply move your partner safely and effectively in the water are necessary. However, the great beauty and freedom of the Watsu Explorer path is its immediacy because it is coming from listening and exploration, not from a sequence or techniques. Sequence and mastering technique is certainly useful for a professional level practitioner, but Explore Flow can be a much more interesting and applicable way of cultivating the spirit of Watsu as a way of life. Professional practitioners may find that the practice of Explore Flow gives new relevance to the sequences that they have mastered, and opens up whole new creative worlds and sensitivity for their work with clients.

Who is interested in Explore Flow will benefit greatly by first opening to perceive what is truly arising and from there will be FREE to explore the resonant flow. Many people, whether beginners or seasoned professionals, can tend to become easily distracted or lose their connection with the "inner dialogue". In the Watsu Explorer Path, we have added the solo "somatic movement meditations" (called Explore Water) to help us perceive the flow within ourselves and learn the art of dialogue with that flow. The dialogue is an interplay between simple listening and somatic response.

Some simple observations that may tune us in to the world of our inner movements and natural flow are:

How do I feel my breath as it exchanges between my inner and outer environments?

Can I feel the weight of my body? The buoyancy?

Can I feel the pulse of my heart?

Do I sense the air or water or clothing on my skin?

When I listen deeply, how does my body naturally want to move and express its organic nature?

These are just simple beginnings, but in the course of an Explore Flow sharing, can provide awareness to bring us back into a space of listening and resonance with our partner(s).

Ultimately, the path of Explore Flow is one of naturalness and simplicity. Anybody can practice and enjoy its pleasures. Life's movements are happening inside of us at all times regardless of whether we notice. Our bodies and hearts are engaged in a process of perceiving the world around us and within us and responding in each moment. When we perceive this flow, we more fully touch our humanness and that of others. We can perceive that below our personalities, our differences of opinion, our varied lifestyle choices, that we are human beings first. We share an ancient heritage, a sacred commonality and great hope for future unity. The flow arrives from the source. We are never separate from the source. The Watsu Explorer path is one way, and a very enjoyable one at that, to know our human connection and future potential more intimately.

THE VITAL IMPORTANCE OF THE PAUSE

When we are engaged in "exploring flow" . . . the great mediator between the In and the Out . . . the expanse and the contract is the PAUSE. It is the non-action from which all action is born, the mother of the flow, the subtle pulsing potentiality that precedes manifestation. To dive into the depths of the Explore Flow path, it is vital that we become intimate friends with the pause . . . as it is here where communion and healing begins.

The Source And The Flow

Like any river or stream of water, the flow is born of a source. Often we do not know the origin of the source. Sometimes in our curiosity, we go seeking the "source". Metaphorically, it may be "underground". It may be frozen in the form of "ice" or high above our heads in a "lofty thunderhead". In searching for the source, sometimes we track "up river". Seeking the source may send it further into refuge. The search for the source can begin and end here and now when we recognize that the source is inherent in the flow. From a systemic point of view, one single drop equals the entire ocean. When we drop into the pause and listen lightly with all of our heart, we can sense the essence, the origin, the latent potentiality from which the flow is born. No amount of seeking will bring us any closer to the source of the flow than we already are right now.

In Watsu and Tantsu this pause (known as "stillness") floats on 'the emptiness that resides at the bottom of the breath." Following our in-breath and our out-breath is one of the most natural ways to know the flow and the pockets of pause inside of the flow. There is no need to change or manipulate your breath to be anything different than it already is. The simple act of noticing your breath helps to create balance and over time any necessary changes in your breathing will happen naturally. Our bodies are a miraculous mélange of intelligent body-mind-emotional intricacy, that when given the right environment, flow naturally towards a state of receptivity and balance. Simple noticing of the breath, simple noticing of ourselves, just as we are, here, right now. . . is the first step in creating that healthy environment. When we slow down into ourselves, we become more sensitive containers for our partner's experience.

Flow Is In Your Nature

Nature flows and fluxes and pauses. Fruits return to the ground after the long summer season to pause (decompose) in the cool moist earth. Seeds rest, pregnant with latent potentiality ready to return to life's growth cycle upon the perfect conditions in the Spring. We too, are magnificent manifestations of the natural world. We too, live in inherent cycles of birth, growth, death, transformation, pause and rebirth. Watsu Tantsu Explore Flow serves as a safe and supported "living laboratory" in which we can accept, live and experiment with life's cyclical nature. A Watsu or Tantsu sharing has cycles of Follow Movement, Explore Movement, Stillness (Pause), just like nature. What we learn inside of a Watsu or Tantsu sharing can then be brought out into how we live our day-to-day lives in resonance with nature's cycles.

The Fear Of The Pause

Our modern society has conditioned us for input and action. We have been trained that if we are not "doing something" that we are lazy or will fall behind or "lose ground." From a neurological perspective, being in constant action is counter-productive.

As the practice of Explore Flow is endless, goal-less or, as Harold says "with no last line", there is no need to try to accomplish or arrive at the end. What's the hurry? No "award" awaits the end of a sequence well executed in the "right" amount of time. In Watsu and Tantsu Explore Flow, the exchange is an experience that validates itself. Enjoy each moment of its luxurious flow. Don't be concerned to "finish". The cycle tends to find it's own "finish" that may or may not look like what you expected. Like this, you will have all the time in the world to "drop into the pause". ENJOY!

The pause is an inherent part of the deep listening process in the practice. It is the rest, the fallow, the re-absorption, the honoring of the latent potentiality, trust in the rhythms of the universe. It takes courage to PAUSE, because our society generally doesn't support this patient inner listening. The pause gives opportunity to listen deeply within oneself. It gives an opportunity to hear the voice of our own Truth. It gives opportunity for vital life force to grow. It gives possibility to expand our perception of the world around us. It allows us to recognize that we can be simultaneously autonomous AND in collaborative sharing with each other. It gives us the incentive to know our own individual organic rhythms FREE from culturally imposed beliefs and mechanized cadences.

How can we really be ourselves if we have not stopped to listen to who we really are? Listen deeply to your hearts desires and your natural rhythms, the callings of your cells, the movement of your fluid. A Watsu or Tantsu sharing gives space and containment for your inner inquiry.

Don't be afraid of silence. The pause need not only be a point along a Watsu or Tantsu progression. Perceive the needs of your partner, and when you sense it . . . you can slow down, open up, be still and let awareness grow in the stillness of the "pause." Be willing to rest in the pause as nourishment for both you and your Watsu or Tantsu companion.

Moments Of Integration

The pause is not falling asleep or just hanging out. The pause is not "stopping"

The pause ("stillness") is light and wide full presence awareness of JUST THE WAY THINGS ARE . . . right now. . . and a personal witnessing of how they pulse, change and evolve. It is the willingness to flow with the change.

Pause equals integration. The movements, contact and sensorial input of a Watsu or Tantsu sharing can introduce a myriad of new neurological information to our nervous systems (whether giver, receiver or witness). This new information enriches and complexifies one's nervous system's capacity to adapt and respond to new situations.

Integration is very important. Once new "information" has been introduced to the nervous system, a period of pause (or stillness) is essential so that our systems have the "time and space" to integrate what it has learned. Without the pause, an information overload can occur. In overload, essentially all systems shut down in a mode of self-protection. All healthy living systems thrive in this cycle of input then integration. On a base level, think about digestion. Imagine that you just eat and eat without pause and never give time for the food you take in to digest. What could have been potential nourishment becomes a toxic overload and our intelligent bio-systems shut down to say "enough". The function is the same with any input to our system, whether food, movement, contact, information, mental process, relationship, etc. All living systems need a balance of input and integration for ultimate health.

As we are all unique, some "systems" integrate more rapidly; others may need more time to absorb. Some need more input, some less. Our objective when sharing Watsu or Tantsu is to remain lovingly open and perceptive to the needs of whom we are holding in our arms, without opinion, without judgment, without imposing our own "schedule" on the other. It is our privilege to hold this fine soul in our arms and help to facilitate their experience.

So, we invite you to simply slow down, notice life happening around you and get used to that long, slow melting into the Pause . . . see what happens! You may be delightfully surprised of all that "occurs" under the busy happenings of every day life . . . life's intricate and subtle movements are so fascinating and we can become intimate with them in the deep listening of the pause. Ahhhh!

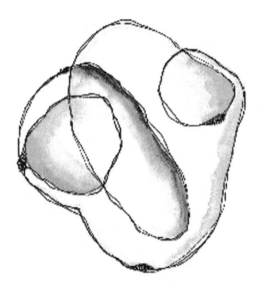

The drawings in this section were made by Ateeka as she watched our first Explorer Path class.

THE PARTICIPATORY WITNESS

The Watsu Tantsu Explorer Path is unique in its use of "triads" during the meditative aquatic and land explorations. The inclusion of a third person to the usual duo creates a new level of trust and connection by diffusing the two-way polarity and opens up to new possibilities of relating with others in a truly evolutionary human way.

This third person is not just an observer; he/she is an essential contribution to the constant flow of energy between the three. This person's witnessing amplifies the resonance of the group and helps to hold the space for the sharing. He/she shifts from simply being an "audience" to becoming a "Participatory Witness" of all life unfolding within the triad's immediate environment. Holding the space means being part of the space.

The participatory witness becomes a part of the event, a part of the happening. As has been proposed in quantum physics research, an observer always affects the reality. True observation invites one to set aside their own personal overlays (emotional charge, opinion, judgment, even agreement) and be in pure witnessing, where one can access pure feeling sense in side their own body, which, in turn gives rise to a greater coherence amongst the three. Simple presence influences, in known or unknown ways, how a Watsu sharing unfolds. All three participants can be in a state of "supported not-knowing", leaving space and infinite possibilities for "magic" to happen.

In Watsu Tantsu Explore Flow, no one role (giver, receiver or witness) is more important than the other. All are flowing equals and all contribute to and benefit from the experience. The participatory witness contributes his/her whole self to the exploration of the triad, supporting and holding the space with his/her own consciousness. It is a sacred role of Presence and connection that creates containment for the receiver's experience of freedom. Interestingly enough however, not only the "receiver" receives because as with all things in the flow of life, what benefits one, benefits all. Watsu Tantsu Explorer sharings are deep experiments in symbiosis.

The participatory witness gives deep relevance to the process happening in their front of their eyes. It is an act of clear witnessing, not voyeurism.

Rather than being "watched", who receives is being "watched over", which is synonymous with feeling safe and contained in a non-threatening and often healing environment. By becoming an active energetic participant, a profound containment for the receiver is created and within this exchange, diffuses the polarity created by two.

The three way mutual reciprocity of the triad creates an environment for clear understanding and diffuses possible projection or identification to the "other". Instead, the triad encourages the development of a direct relationship with the Infinite . . . one that need not pass through any other human or any particular system or technique. The addition of the participatory witness allows the "personalities" of those sharing to take the back seat, and allows the spontaneous "flow" to become the primary focus of the sharing. Felt sensations of gratitude, deep peace, joy, pleasure and sense of community are facilitated by this sharing in three.

The human nervous system is enriched by new and varied information and the participatory witness helps to facilitate the healthy assimilation of "new information" to the receiver's system. Physiologically, all participants in a sharing benefit. The profound sharing increases the adaptability of one's nervous system, strengthens the immune system and reduces stress and its related physiological indicators. Clearly, exploration in the triad amplifies the potential for the containment of Watsu and Tantsu as a deeply healing and meditative practice.

Being in the role of the participatory witness has a value added benefit. It helps one to develop a capacity for increased sensitivity and perception of the world around them, to become more empathetic of what others might be feeling, to sense one's own subtle inner currents of life. One can learn to become consciously interactive with "the field." Any interaction that one has, any movement one does, any thought that occurs comes from an immense body of vibratory information that is often referred to as "the field." It is a collective reservoir of all that has ever happened and all that ever will, of all that is possible and all that may come to pass. The "field" gestates infinite possibilities. Humans have the conscious power to bring certain possibilities to life. In the role of participatory witness, one can practice and hone their skills of perception due to the "passive" role. One can inquire into the felt sensations in their own physical heart, or how the breath of all 3 in the triad moves in the direction of coherency. We may be able to "see", with a soft peripheral gaze, very subtle movements spawning it the receiver's body when in the phase of Stillness. These are all recognitions of the other that serve to help us recognize our own true essence more clearly.

Trust, connection, increased sensitivity, profound containment are all enhanced with the addition of the participatory witness in the Watsu and Tantsu sharings. It is rare to find a practice this simple that can bring about such deep listening, heart felt communication and peace. Watsu Tantsu Explore Flow offers an opportunity to live this way within its sharings, which certainly affects the culture of peace that we are seeking to create. The most minute actions affect the largest scale . . . we start with this. . . the simple and loving containment and connection in three.

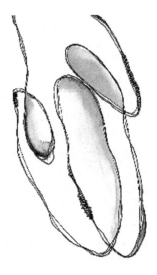

PLAY, HUMOR AND PLEASURE: THE WAY A BODY LEARNS

When do we stop learning? Hopefully never! Introduce into your life new information, new ideas, new movement, new people, new ways of being and you will continue to feel full of vitality and curiosity. Nearly all levels of our being, physical, intellectual, emotional, psychological, neurological, are nourished by encounters with what is innovative and fresh.

So, if learning keeps us so young, vital and alive, why do so many resent the learning process? Our western paradigm for education has been one that generally does not stimulate creativity nor encourage us to be innovative. The institutional education model that most of us have grown up with is one that follows the industrial concept of "accountability" and "control". Fun and creativity take a back seat (or get no seat at all!) to productivity. In this model, motivation suffers and stress increases. It is not a system that encourages growth and renewal. It is not sustainable and will not create a long lasting healthy environment.

Well, artists, rockers and rebels, REJOICE . . . because the path of Core Watsu and Tantsu Explorer goes beyond the institutional rules and gives us a new model for innovative, integrated learning. We play, we laugh, we make contact, we empathize and above all, we enjoy! In the process, we become enriched both individually and on a community level. This is how we truly learn. . . we absorb "information" and transform it, through experience, into personal wisdom.

We Play

"*Play is the exultation of the possible.*" *Martin Buber*

Play is the most primary and fundamental activity that fosters learning and growth. Children intuitively learn through "playing". It is their "job" to play all day, and an important job it is . . . because they are growing in every way at blazing speeds. Animals, in their own unique ways, play their whole lives through. We too can reclaim our right to play! Play is made up of the cycles of free choice, movement and discovery. Core Watsu and Tantsu Explorer is a forum for play and discovery. The phase of EXPLORE FLOW in the progression invites us to develop a presence-filled curiosity and we allow ourselves to be sensitively inquisitive and engaged deeply in the process unfolding before our very eyes and heart. With delight, we can participate in the co-creation of movement expressions of the Watsu or Tantsu sharing.

Engaged play supports healthy development of sense of self and self-esteem. Our sense of humor is born of play. We learn about ourselves, about our own humanity and about how to accept success and make mistakes as a part of an on-going process. When we are well established in our own personal presence, we can be of greater support to another as their process unfolds. This is a fundamental quality that is both learned and utilized in a Watsu or Tantsu sharing. The more present I am in my own being, the more we can both enjoy our shared being-ness in the practice. Play gives rise to coherence.

We Laugh

"*Humor is the affectionate communication of insight.*" *Leo Rosten*

Humor is one of the most important factors in creating a positive emotional state-of-being. In turn, positive emotions create a fertile environment for cognitive and neurological development. Humor is one of the most essential ingredients for integrated learning. A sympathetic glance at the soft side of humanity can bring a kind smile to our face, and a feeling in our cells, that "we are all in this together!" Well-intentioned humor can create a strong bond between us and develop trust. When we are having fun, we generally do not feel under threat. Our nervous system lets down its vigilant guard and a new level of trust and group interaction and synergy arises. Fun leads to trust, and trust tells our systems that it is safe to assimilate new ideas and information.

Emotional intelligence is the ability to perceive and empathize with our own emotions and those of others. As we grew, if we were lucky to have humor and wisdom in our families, we may have learned ways of expressing and embodying the wide range of emotions felt by humans. Others may have learned ways of managing, repressing or using emotions to manipulate the world around us. The heart resonance generated in a Core Watsu or Tantsu sharing offers a possibility to shed new light on our emotions and reclaim our emotional bodies. When peppered with kind and loving humor, this process can become fun, light and penetrate deeper into our heart, than would a forceful catharsis.

Laughing has been scientifically proven to relieve stress and increases vital energy. It creates movement all throughout the body, frees the diaphragm, increases breath capacity and reduces conflict. If two people with opposing viewpoints can find a bridge through humor and laughter, maybe they are not so far away from resolution after all. Humor and laughter facilitates creativity, even in problem solving. When we are resolving conflict, we are opening to new ways, which again, means that our systems are learning something new.

The water in which we practice Watsu is a very resonate element. You may notice when you are in a sharing group, that some silly little human happening sets someone to laugh, and before you know it, the whole pool is in a belly laugh. The water enhances this effect (but it certainly happens on land too!) For years we have heard about the "heart-body-wave" of Watsu. . . maybe now it is time for the "belly-body-laugh-wave." Try it as one of your Watsu experiments. Lightheartedly, find something to get the laughter going, something silly, something common and human . . . and see what happens! The whole pool, the whole room, your whole being will be filled with a bubbly presence of joy and exhilaration. This is a state that education consultant, Mary K. Morrison calls "humergy". A peak moment when you are overflowing with the feeling of vitality, alertness, joy and energy through humor! Humergy is a radically healing state and VERY VERY FUN! I bet you are smiling just reading this right now!

We Empathize

Healthy imitation leads to possibility leads to authenticity.

The act of witnessing a new kind movement in another creates new neurological growth within our own systems. Simply watching another's movement inspires a "kinesthetic empathy" of subtle motor and neural activity in the body. Often we don't even know that a movement, or thought or concept is even possible until we witness it in another. The "Mirror Neuron Theory" suggests that in the act of observation, our bodies empathize with and learn about the movements and gestures we are exposed to.

So, especially in learning new movement, or un-learning repetitive movement patterns, somatic imitation may be a great jump-start. As children we have all learned by imitation, and then as we have matured hopefully taken that inspiration on towards our own authentic expression. The objective is not to "copy" what we have seen but simply have exposure to new possibilities and let our bio-systems take it from there. To try to copy will shut down your creative flow, and inhibit an intelligent organic learning process. Instead a somatic imitation happens simply and automatically, trust that it is happening, sense what the movement might feel like and then just let go. The Core Watsu and Tantsu triad experience offer a great opportunity for learning through this "kinesthetic empathy" as we will sometimes be in the role of the participatory witness. While it may seem that our main "function" is to hold the space for who is receiving, we at the same time receive millions of information impulses every second as we perceive the movement experience our partners. It is learning through empathy and without effort.

When we shift to the role of "giver," our objective is not to imitate what we have witnessed, but the empathetic effects remain imprinted in our tissues and we may find that we can flow through new movements with more ease and grace simply from observing. Out of this new "neural dexterity" can grow new potentials for creative response and authenticity that may not have been possible before. Coupled with other integrative learning tools of play, humor and pleasure, somatic imitation can be very useful in the moment.

We Enjoy

In all of our Watsu and Tantsu sharings, we encourage an atmosphere of ease, enjoyment and pleasure. **Play, humor and empathy evoke ease.** Ease is the opposite of stress and sets the tone for the body's innate regenerative processes to engage naturally. In a pleasure state (when the nervous system is in a state of parasympathetic response), we slow down, cells renew, breathing becomes more ample and relaxed, we notice and enjoy more, and all life processes become more efficient. Pleasure is inherent in the cellular and systemic regenerative processes.

Change, even from a redundant or unhealthy environment to a more positive one can be a stressor to the bio-system if not made with the intention of creating a pleasurable experience. A pleasurable environment gently dissolves negative biological response without aggression. Pleasure paves the way for the nervous system and all of the body's tissues and fluids to be re-informed with new possibilities and a creates a positive biological response in the process of the change. Who is in our Watsu or Tantsu cradle understands that we are here as a friendly support, we are not a threat. In this non-threatening, pleasurable environment, our partner has the opportunity for his/her habitual defensive reactions to transform into positive intention for change. Pleasure is the original alchemist, it transforms!

It is important to understand that pleasure is not "excitement" as is commonly inferred. A stimulating experience can be "sensually pleasurable" and positively invigorating. Exciting events can activate the sympathetic nervous system in a positive way and energizing way. This can be a playful and essential jump-start for igniting more vital life force energy in our systems. However, for the regenerative processes and parasympathetic nervous system mode of repose to be engaged, pleasure is experienced like a wide, vast, expansive sensation of wellbeing, relaxed and being in the flow of life.

As we understand and apply the psycho-somatic importance of pleasure in our sharings, not only does our Watsu or Tantsu companion receive increased benefit, but our energy and creativity also becomes more ample.

We Embody

"A wise man has no extensive knowledge; He who has extensive knowledge is not a wise man." Lao-Tzu - Tao te Ching

When we can truly embody our experiences of play, pleasure, humor, contact, breathing and witnessing, our learning becomes integrated. The combination of all that we have "learned" and our own unique life experience is expressed through us as individuals, not just walking encyclopedias of accumulated knowledge. Learning becomes embodied understanding when it originates from an attitude of playfulness and joy, not obligation or repetitive studying. Learning, practicing, sharing, assimilation, integration of knowledge becomes personal understanding.

Nothing is more boring that someone who simply recites facts. Instead, the fascinating human is the one who simply and honestly lives what they have experienced, and without pretense, remains open to each new adventure. Without play, we become old. Without humor, we become grumpy. Without empathy, we become stuck and rigid. Without pleasure, we become brittle and dry. Jump into the school of life and its ongoing course of "play-sure" (play + pleasure) where you will be most authentically informed and enriched. Dare to dance the juicy dance of life! You might think you look silly . . . but then again, you might make someone smile and that is the start of a wonderful education!

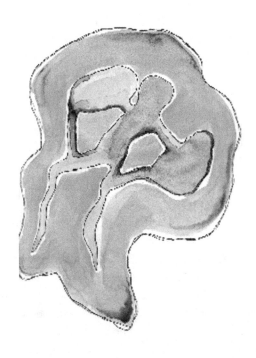

THE REGENERATIVE POTENTIAL OF WATSU AND TANTSU

What is often vaguely referred to as "healing" can more specifically be referred to as "the regenerative process". Living beings have an inherent response towards life. And life itself is always in natural cycles of regeneration which includes letting go of the old and accepting in the new. Each one of us, without effort, is an "autonomous healer". Without our conscious thought, our bodies regenerate themselves daily by calling upon undifferentiated matter in the cellular matrix to take form as differentiated (purpose specific) cells perpetuating the cycle of life. Fetuses "miraculously" grow to be infants and then adults through the completely natural process of regeneration.

Illness and disease arise when our natural inclination towards life, regeneration, is impeded. Long-standing stressful situations and traumatic experiences stored in the body's tissues can compromise the adaptive and varied response of the bio-system needed to be in a vital and healthy state.

Our capacity for regeneration depends greatly upon the environment in which we create for ourselves to live in. Environment is more than the physical place that we happen to find ourselves in, or a simple state of mind. Our environment is determined by how we, consciously or unconsciously, organize and interact with the world around us.

The regenerative process happens naturally in an environment of positive biological response characterized by easeful pleasure and openness. Cells regenerate when the nervous system is in an open and unthreatened state of parasympathetic repose. This environment is physiologically recognized by a slower heart beat, relaxed respiration, undilated pupils, pink skin, active digestion, sweet breath and more. The regenerative processes are extremely efficient and do not require great amounts of energy to function. They do, however, require a positive and supportive environment in which to function.

When in an environment of threat or danger, one must allocate all of his or her available energy to defend against the aggressor. In this "vigilant" state, the bio-system's priority is to survive rather than regenerate. Regenerative processes temporarily take a back seat to an implicit defense response. This environment of defense is physiologically recognized by a rapid heartbeat, shallow respiration, dilated pupils, profuse perspiration, pallid skin, blood flow towards the body's limbs and away from digestive processes and more. When in actual danger, it is very important to the body to have the capacity to respond in this way.

Unfortunately, the fast paced demands of today's world create an overdose of stress and tension for most people. The nervous system perceives this "accelerated rhythm" as a dangerous aggressor and reacts biologically as if it were in great danger. Many people in today's busy world remain in an "on alert" energy-consuming survival mode than in an energy-efficient regenerative rest mode. In either case, one can choose to manage their reactions or responses to create a more life-affirming environment around them.

To generate health, one chooses to create an appropriate environment to activate the regenerative process. Obviously one cannot "command" the body to relax and let go. That may cause even more agitation and stress to the system. However, through the practices of Watsu and Tantsu, one can shift from "react" to "relax" so that he/she may have a glance of previously unexperienced environments for health.

The first objective is to create a positive, supportive and unthreatening environment. The intention is cultivate a new space for enhanced perception and ultimately, change. The practice is approached with humanness, with hearts open and with eyes on the wholeness of potential for health.

Watsu and Tantsu are ideal practices for re-initiating the regenerative processes.

The containment of Watsu and Tantsu create a safe place where one can experiment with change with the physical and energetic support of a partner or group. The holds and cradles of Watsu and Tantsu grant the opportunity to return to a protected neutral environment, like a mother's womb, where all creation begins.

In Watsu, the warm water further enhances this environment of simultaneous containment and creation as well as offering a constant sensorial pleasure to the skin. The diversity of the body's relationship with gravity that is experienced in the water gives new opportunities for efficiently changing and opening to new environment options.

Both Watsu and Tantsu have the potential as processes for listening deeply to one's own inner movement. As one learns to perceive and engage in the creative movement of life, he/she help oneself and fellow companions on this path to slow down and experience wholeness and potentiality. Following the expression of one's own organic movement rather than mindlessly "doing a sequence", honors personal rhythms and helps to develop a relationship of trust and collaboration between human beings. After this natural movement has been followed and explored, all action eventually returns to "stillness". Watsu and Tantsu observe these moments of stillness with quiet holds. Holds create coherence and connection between the persons involved and return both (or all in the case of work in triads) to the "place" of creation, where the everyday miracle of regenerative processes re-ignite naturally without effort and with ease.

Certainly Watsu and Tantsu are not the only practices that activate the processes of regeneration, but when practiced with non-repetitive, sensitive presence, can be a very effective path of change for health, wholeness and happiness.

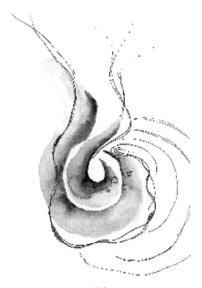

NEURAL NETWORKS OF INTELLIGENCE

Our Three "Brains" and the Nervous System
Excerpt from **Love Is Under My Skin**: *Explorations in Systemic Yoga* by Ateeka

Our primary "centers of intelligence" are the brain, the heart and the gastrointestinal tract. Each of these centers has a very large concentration of neurons and neural activity that relate intrinsically with our perception of the world around us and how the nervous system responds.

The nervous system is essentially a electro-corporeal web of symbiotic relationships. Although anatomically, our nervous system is made of cellular matter and organic proteins, its true "living" aspect is the exchange of information and responses to the stimuli that it constantly receives.

Traditionally, the entirety of the autonomic nervous system has been understood by differentiating it into specific "systems" with specific functions. New research rooted in ancient wisdom helps us to understand the nervous system instead as a vibrant web of inter-related electro-magnetic impulses, messages and responses to stimuli

Each aspect of the autonomic nervous system has unique qualities each forming a "center of intelligence" that senses, perceives, responds and interacts. Traditional Chinese medicine has long suggested that the human body has three "brains", not just one! Available to perceive and respond to information are the cranial brain, the heart brain and the gut or gastro-intestinal brain. All are made up of large concentrations of nerve ganglia . As our methods of measuring electro-magnetic activity become more sophisticated, science is beginning to recognize and validate this ancient theory as true.

The Three "Brains"

The enteric nervous system (ENS) thrives within the gastro-intestinal tract and has the vital role of sensing personal safety and nourishment. It is home to our inherent sense of "knowing." This neural network forms the "gut" brain and is our primary level of perception of stimuli.

The parasympathetic nervous system (PNS) with its primary nerves running from the base of the brain to the sacrum is a reservoir of life force energy. When our system is in balance, it serves as a connection to an infinite source of undifferentiated energy, of potentiality, the ground from which our actions arise and return into. Cellular regeneration and healing occurs when the body is in a parasympathetic mode. While this neural network is distributed widely throughout the entire body, we find a dense concentration of nerve cells in the heart that serve to perceive the "weather" of our personal environment. This could be thought of as the "heart brain".

The sympathetic nervous system (SNS) is the active mode of choice, curiosity, individuality and expression. It also is the system that responds actively to threatening situations. It's primary nerves originate and expand outward from nerve ganglia in the thoracic and lumbar regions of the spine. We can associate this system with the "cranial brain" and its innate capacity to process and respond to millions of incoming information impulses every second.

Essentially, the "gut" senses and feels, the heart perceives and the brain processes and acts.

The "information" sensed, perceived and communicated by this intricately woven nervous system can be described as an ever-widening field of infinite combinations of electromagnetic impulses, exchanging within environments of varying densities and gravities and other energetic factors. The exchange of information never ceases to exist. It is always in movement. Living organisms thrive in an environment of constant change and exchange, where information re-informs, complexifies and strengthens the adaptability of neural network. As the old adage says, "use it or lose it." New information presented in a creative, pleasurable environment thrills the nervous system.

Why then, do some people seem to be more perceptive to the world around them? Why do others seem callous and inattentive to their place in the world? What we have been sensitized to perceive and what we have been conditioned not to perceive depends largely on our culture and environment. Most religions, governments, educational systems and cultural norms have trained us to follow a doctrine, dogma or set of regulations rather than to trust our cellular wisdom. One widely used, yet dangerous catch-word in Western advertising has been "convenient". Services of convenience have numbed our nervous system's ancient sensing and perceptive qualities and have made us to rely more and more only on repetitive schemes conditioned into the nervous system over time. This unbalance in the exchange of the various aspects of the nervous system has rendered us more susceptible to disease and control . For example, the convenience of buying any vegetable that we "want" at any season of the year at one mega-grocery store is a convenience that has desensitized our system to "know" what foods are nutritious and most useful for us. We have become run by our cravings rather than by perception. It is easy to control a population that is discouraged to sense, perceive or choose their own actions, and all who wish to be in power over others know that.

The origins of our nervous systems have evolved over millions of years of information input and biological response. How we have evolved as a species has been determined by the intrinsic interaction of the three "brains" as they exchanged with environmental information. We all have the power to widen and sensitize the spectrum of our sensing and perceiving capabilities when we are willing to soften into a wide and restful parasympathetic state more of the time. We now have the possibility to choose and guide our biological responses to be positive, life-affirming states of choice and response, rather than control and reaction.

Underlying the entirety of this neural net of intelligence is the fluid system of our bodies. It bathes, floats, nourishes, supports and is a messenger of resonant information throughout the system. Fluid faithfully retains and remembers the frequency of any information that it is exposed to. It amplifies and accelerates any electromagnetic impulses of the nervous system. The fluid coursing within us mediates the interactions between the intelligence centers of the gut, the heart and the brain.

Enteric Nervous System
A Sense of Safety

The enteric nervous system (ENS) is an ancient neural network of sensing/feeling intelligence and is our most immediate connection with primordial aspects of ourselves. Embedded in the lining of the gastrointestinal tract, over 100 million neurons (1/1000th of that of the human brain) as well as neurotransmitters and proteins make up the enteric circuit that acts independently, learns, remembers and detects the underlying "safety" of any given situation.

Our primordial call to feel "safe in our own skin" is closely related to nourishment and "having enough". Millions of years ago, the first animals to inhabit Earth were simple tubular forms of life that attached themselves to rocks or plants and waited for "food" to pass by. They developed primitive tube-like nervous systems that met their needs for taking in nourishment and expelling excess.

As life evolved, higher animals and eventually humans developed more complex nervous systems, allowing them to reproduce and seek nourishment. Still, the primordial presence of the enteric nervous system has endured over millions of years and is present and fundamental in modern humans.

It is fascinating to note that in early embryonic development, an undifferentiated mass of tissue called the neural crest initiates the growth of the nervous system. One part of this mass eventually differentiates to become the central nervous system (later differentiating into the spinal cord with cranial nerves and more) and the other part migrates downward to become the enteric nervous system in the gut. Much later in the fetal stages, the vagus nerve develops and connects the nerve networks. The development in the womb is like a fast forward replay of all evolution over time. It is when we emerge from the womb that we have the opportunity for the next step in conscious creation of the future of our species.

On Knowing

Despite having highly complex nervous systems, the enteric remains our primary sensor of safety and nourishment. Through an instinctive "feeling sense," the primordial enteric system optimally detects what is appropriate for us to ingest, both physically and energetically, how to assimilate it and how to expel excess. The primal intelligence of this "gut brain" embodies a sense of "knowing". By listening to the "messages" of our "gut feelings" we can know whether an outside influence is of assistance/support or is of aggression.

Many illnesses of the gastrointestinal tract can be traced to chronic tension of the enteric nervous system. We, as humans, need to feel safe, nurtured and nourished first and foremost, and then we can move on to more refined curiosities/investigations. If, we find ourselves in an environment of danger or lack, the intelligence of the enteric system will alert the sympathetic nervous system to respond or react. With the stimulation overload and "conveniences" of the modern age, humans (especially those of industrialized cultures) tend to have lost their capacity for "knowing" and rely on outside sources to inform (or often misinform) them of the nature of a situation.

A very simple example: when determining whether milk is consumable, most people now look at the expiration date on the carton to guide their decision. Instinctively, however, even after checking the date (rational mind) , most people will then smell the milk (enteric system impulse). Inhaling a sour odor creates an immediate response on part of the enteric nervous system that inform us not to ingest the milk. If you pay attention you can even feel the tissues of the stomach contract. Why is it necessary to have the printed date when our own systems inform us with much more immediacy and efficiency?

Animals and indigenous people still have this sense well developed and as we learn to trust our own system more inherently, we will guide ourselves towards situations and environments that enhance our wellbeing rather than engaging in defense or aggression. Learning to perceive and honor the "feeling in the gut" is the first step towards taking responsibility for our livelihoods.

The Parasympathetic Nervous System
A Wide Sense of Place

The parasympathetic nervous system is the state of repose and regeneration in our system. It nurtures the qualities of inner awareness and introspection, receptive involution and gestation of the new. It is essentially a space of potentiality, where new information is perceived and integrated.

Researchers at the Heartmath Institute in Boulder, Colorado have done extensive studies into the neural network of the heart. They have discovered that the heart has a complex intrinsic nervous system allowing it to act independently of the cranial brain. This "heart brain" is highly sensitive to the electromagnetic frequencies of other living beings, especially human beings. The "heart brain" could be responsible for perceiving up to 80% of incoming information from the outside world and the communication of it to the cranial brain primarily through the vagus nerve. It has been discovered that the heart is not simply a pump that serves to move blood through our circulatory system, but of equal importance, the neural network of the heart serves to balance, harmonize and synchronize cognitive, emotional and physiological processes. When all are in balance, it is referred to as a state of "coherence" (resonant frequency). Feelings of love and gratitude and empathy serve to strengthen this coherence.

Coherency in the "heart brain" evokes a parasympathetic response of wellness, peace, connection and "sense of place" in which we exist. When the system is in a parasympathetic state we feel contained in spaciousness where the regenerative processes can take place. Human beings have an innate instinct to seek for a sense of place. The system at rest is a system that has oriented itself, has a sense of place in the grand scheme of things and receives vast nourishment from energetic sources. When the system is at rest, energy is acquired rather than consumed and the body can regenerate new cells and more easily expel waste.

The parasympathetic nervous system responds to slowing down, perceiving more and returning to the awareness of our inner selves. It is enhanced by positive thought, interaction with nature, creative expression, caring human touch and the presence of healthy, loving relationships in our lives. Parasympathetic dominance creates an environment for health, healing and renewal.

The Sympathetic Nervous System
A Sense of Self

Curiosity, choice and individual expression define the healthy functioning of the sympathetic nervous system. The actions determined by the SNS direct our inner awareness outward in either personal expression or vigilance. Healthy responses and subsequent actions of the sympathetic nervous system are our links to community, a reaching outward to know ourselves in relationship to the world around us. We come to know and define who we are through the reflection of others.

A basic human drive is to explore the space around itself. The sympathetic nervous system supports this drive as it is action and exploration oriented. The alertness of this state can be expressed either in expansive clarity (response) or defensive alarm (reaction).

The alarm aspect of sympathetic nervous system reacts with an ancient protection instinct. When faced with a threat (physical, emotional or other) the system reacts with either fighting, escaping or "freezing" (in humans, immobilization of the breath), all of which create an intense stress on the physiological body. The priority of the blood flow rushes to the periphery of the body, heart rate speeds up and the hormones of adrenaline and cortisol are released into the blood stream. Active biological processes are accelerated in order to facilitate the fight, flight or freeze. The defense reaction plays a vital role during the immediate moments of stress/trauma, it may in fact, save one's life. However, the amount of constant stressors in our modern daily life have rendered most human systems out of balance, with the sympathetic alarm reaction taking precedence even when life-threatening conditions do not exist. Modern business models have capitalized on the "imprintability" of the nervous system by creating subtle constant currents of fear and stress within our society in order to dis-empower the individual and benefit economically just a few at the top at the power structure. Governments and businesses collaborate with media channels to weave stories making us believe that we are always under a threat of attack (terrorism), or lack (economic crisis) or harm (avian flu). This state of constant stress and disconnection from a more natural rhythm of life contributes to an overactive sympathetic nervous system and is the cause most of the health problems that we encounter today.

It is interesting to note that exists have a fourth type of sympathetic reaction to "dangerous" situations, the "taking care" reaction. It is more frequently seen in women. When faced with undue stress, one may deeply suppress their dissatisfaction and appear to shoulder all of the responsibility. The type that displays this reaction to stress may seem to be "in control of it all" and is often even admired for this by the others around her. The outer appearance of calm, however, can be a façade as she has ingested the stress deep inside her system. What has been suppressed will eventually need to exit the system. Often years and years of ingested stress makes itself evident in chronic or life-threatening illness.

Making Changes

Although most Western medical theory has led us to believe that the autonomic nervous system functioning is automatic and cannot be regulated, we now can take responsibility for the balance of our system's responses through various methods of meditation, movement, breathing, Systemic Yoga, Watsu, Tantsu, bio-feedback and self care. We can become more aware of the "environments" that we have created in our lives and whether they are beneficial or harmful to our health.

At a natural and unstressed rhythm, we can change the factors that cause disharmony in our lives. The input of new and fresh situations and experiences and stimuli will help to resensitize and complexify the response of the nervous system and empower us towards taking care of our own health and happiness.

It is important to remember the sympathetic and parasympathetic systems are mutual and supportive. Both have positive biological responses and can be pushed towards imbalance resulting in negative biological response. Our systems thrive in a diverse environment of action and rest, inner dwelling and outer expression. Health, physiological, emotional and mental, depends largely on the awareness and balance of the interactions of the various aspects of the autonomic nervous system.

AUTONOMIC NERVOUS SYSTEM CHARACTERISTICS	
PARASYMPATHETIC	SYMPATHETIC (in stressful situation)
Repose / Regeneration	Alertness / Activity / Alarm
Acquisition and conservation of energy	Expenditure of energy
Blood flow towards digestive tract	Blood flow towards skeletal muscles
Pink and dry skin (peripheral vasodilation)	Pallid & cold sweaty skin (vasoconstriction)
Support of organ function	Support of movement/action
Heart rate slower/functions with less effort	Heart Rate Faster/Tachycardia
Enhanced immune system functioning	Decrease of immune system functioning
Originates in cranial & sacral nerve ganglia	Originates in thoracic & lumbar nerve ganglia
Supports central circulation / venous flow	Supports peripheral circulation/arterial flow
Muscular relaxation	Muscular tension and rigidity
Pupils constrict – less light enters eyes	Pupils dilate – more light enters eyes
More saliva secretion/moist mouth	Saliva secretion decreases/dry mouth
Stomach secretions increase	Adrenaline secretion increase
Bronchioles (lungs) constrict	Bronchioles dilate
Improved metabolism & use of oxygen	Less availability of oxygen to cells
Better hemostatia (blood clotting)	Decreased hemostatia
Intestinal mobility increased	Intestinal mobility decreased
Colon empties	Colon retains contents
Bladder empties	Bladder delays emptying
	SYMPATHETIC (in active but unstressful situation)
Condensing and involuting	Expanding and unfolding
	Alertness/Activity
	Utilization of Energy

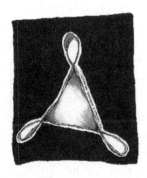
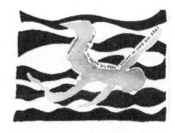

HOME SPA WATSU

Since home spas (such as those made by Jacuzzi) are more common than warm pools, I developed Home Spa Watsu to make Watsu more accessible. The seats in a home spa allow the practitioner to sit in a way that frees all four limbs to hold and work with a person. Though this can be adapted to any model spa, the ideal is one large enough to float someone with a simple bench around the inside. Half the moves are done with someone lying across our knees, his or her head supported in a comfortable head cradle that allows movement, and out of which the head can be easily lifted to move the receiver into other positions. Make a head cradle by slipping pipe insulation foam over and around the edge of a leaf skimmer and tying it to the handle. The handle (without a pole) is then tied in a way that it hangs over the edge of the pool. The foam covered rim and skimmer webbing provide perfect support for the head. The temperature of the Home Spa should be kept under 99 Fahrenheit during a session.

Home Spa Watsu has become a new form of aquatic bodywork in its own right. The flow of Watsu is mitigated, but the practitioner's stable position facilitates stronger stretches and bodywork than can be done in an open pool. Its firmer holding provides a safe boundary within which people can go deeper into themselves. Many receivers who had previously received pool Watsu have contrasted this deeper internal state they access in Home Spa Watsu with the greater outward expansiveness they had experienced in a larger pool, finding a unique value in each.

Floating someone across your legs there is a greater access to the back, to work it from below, and to work it from both sides, than on land. When I gave a session to someone who used to be a trainer for the Dallas Cowboys, he immediately saw its value for athletes. When I gave a session to someone who works with children she saw its value in homes of children with special conditions. We are training Practitioners to train families in its simpler moves. Watsu Practitioners with training in Zen Shiatsu and/or Tantsu can use it professionally.

Watsu is Zen Shiatsu taken into the water. Tantsu is the return of Watsu onto the land. Home Spa is the return of Tantsu into the water. On this shore, in these amphibious shallows, with all this coming and going, whatever you learn in water and on land converge.

Stay centered throughout, dropping deeper into that center at the bottom of each breath. Just as we start each session with hands on the heart and body center of the other, it is maintaining the open connection of these two within ourselves that is the foundation of our work. Stay open hearted throughout, letting whatever energy rises, rise up through the heart. This is the foundation for being with another without any kind of intention, a level of being which allows the other to access the deepest foundations of their own self-healing.

Many receivers speak of perceiving a profound sense of oneness. As a giver I have always felt that this oneness is our oneness with everything. It is one of the most powerful forms of meditation that I know. The more a giver can work this close and stay centered, the more both giver and receiver can avoid transference or attachment.

Because most of the time the practitioner works from a sitting position, the places where he sits in relationship to the receiver are defined as consecutive posts in the following.

First Post

This first post, alongside the chest, is the best to begin almost every session. The containment achieved by holding one side and working up from the other supports the receiver's perception of the body being worked on as a whole rather than in parts. Besides reducing the kind of resistance that occurs when one part is focused on, including the resistance caused by the receiver trying to help reduce the tension in that part, this being worked on from both sides, increases the receiver's sense of the unity of his or her body, and because we are breathing together and working so close to the heart, the unity of heart, body and mind.

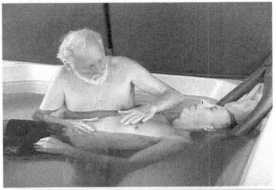

Begin by having the receiver lay across your legs with the head supported at the occiput by a head cradle. Rest one hand lightly on the body center, below the navel, and the other on the heart center. Connect your breathing, and, as you both breath out, rock gently into the two centers. When you feel the breath coming in lifting your hands, breathe in rocking back. Continue for several breaths.

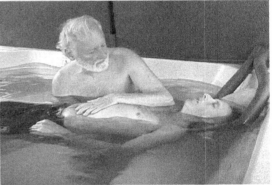

Leave one hand on a center and reach up under the back with the other. Stay connected with the breath. Work up into the musculature on each side of the spine from underneath. Lift up with pointed fingers, or grip and squeeze and shake. Work freely. Return both hands to the centers as often as feels right. And return to work up under the back with one or the other hand as often as feels right. The warmth of the water, and its removal of gravity's pressure on the spine, and the kind of movement that is possible even in this limited amount in water, can make this more effective than most bodywork on land. Let the tempo change freely, stillness, or still moves, following the more active one.

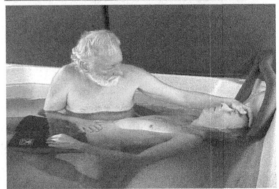

Explore how far up into the shoulder and neck you can comfortably reach and work. Explore what can be done at this post when you reach across the body and pull up into the back… and how the hand on the front can explore, coordinating its placement, movement and pressure with the hand pulling up from underneath, and release the stored tension in the structures between them.

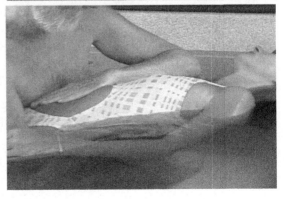

Second Post

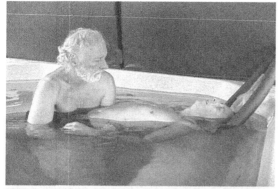

Sit alongside the lower back, the top of the legs over your right thigh, the back resting on the other. This is a post where we can effectively work the lumbar and hips. We can also bring the receiver up into a sitting position at this post, being careful to not let the neck hyperextend, and firmly clasp them with both our legs and our arms. Using our legs to clasp and hold frees our arms to work with the body. The shoulder is accessible and an upward rotation can be very effective in this position. We can also shake some movement into the arm and hand. We can stretch back the arm and work under the shoulder blade, sliding it gently over our extended fingers with the outbreath. We can hold both arms stretched back and rock with the breath.

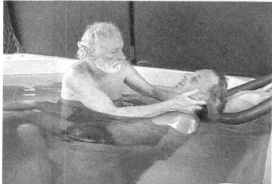

We can alternate gently pulling one shoulder forward and pushing the other back opening the chest.

We can press and hold the far leg to the shoulder, rocking with the breath. Having the bench under us and a wall behind makes it easier for us to hold powerful stretches such as this one pulling the whole leg up.

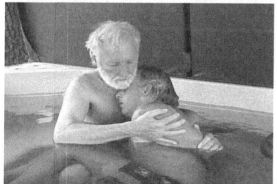

Our seated position allows us full use of both our legs and arms. Our feet can comfortably hook and hold a leg out. When we find ourselves comfortably holding someone in a powerful stretch like this, we can then explore whatever gentle movement or rocking might add to its effect. In this post we are still close enough to the heart center that one hand can, when called, return to rest on it.

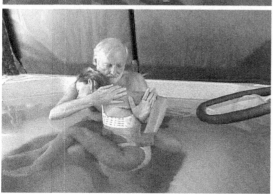
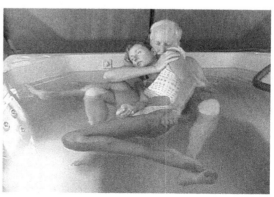

Whenever it feels drawn there, the hand on the heart center can move up to rest on the mind center.

Having a bench in the pool gives us a place to raise one leg and support someone over it, freeing both our hands to work. They can access the neck at the same time we are press stretching the propped leg. Sitting comfortably on the bench against the wall facilitates a continuous movement with the four limbs out from the center, coordinating stretches, pointwork and joint mobilization with full body movement in ways, and with an ease, that would be impossible to duplicate on land. At the same time holding the other to our heart center helps facilitate the kind of synchronization of brain and body rhythms or waves with our heart's rhythms that research finds essential for true emotional healing.

After focusing on the neck we can lay the person back and rock them for a moment. We can then return the head to the head cradle.

Stretches should be gradually arrived at and held without any intense rocking. There can be a gentle pulsing. Before any session, you should determine if there are any problems with the back, neck, shoulder, hip or any other structures and adapt your session accordingly. Ask what positions, stretches or moves that they know exasperate the problems in those areas and avoid them. Insist that they give you feedback and do not persist with any action causing discomfort.

These moves are a sequence that must be learned, but ways of exploring what can be effective and appropriate from each of the places, or posts, a spa presents.

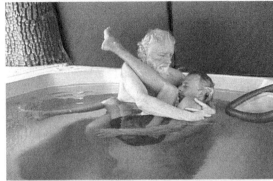
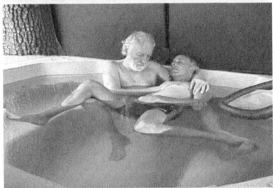
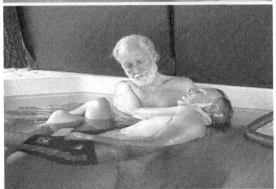
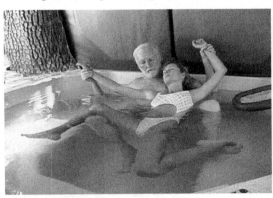
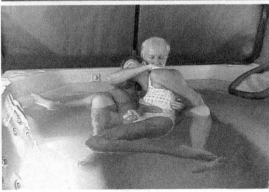

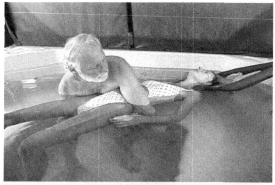

Move further down with the knees over your right thigh and the sacrum over your left. With your partner's head back in the head cradle, explore what bodywork can be done with the hip and the near leg.

Starting at the top of the leg, we can reach all the way around it with one arm, our hand getting a grip on the outside of the near hip, avoiding any contact that would be inappropriate or invasive. The other arm can reach around the waist to brace the tugging of the near leg. Be careful to tug the leg toward the foot not out to the side.

After tugging at the hip, we can rest the near leg over our knee and roll the leg gradually working towards the foot. Instead of grasping the leg roll it with an open hand, pushing with the heel of your hand and pulling from the opposite side with your fingertips allowing the leg to roll freely and release tension at the hip.

Points around the knee could also be worked on from this and the following posts.

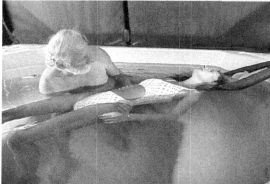

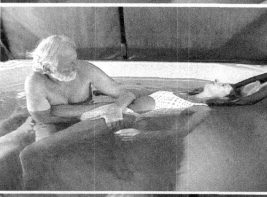

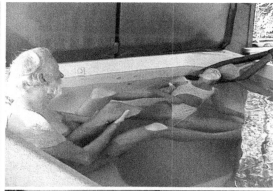

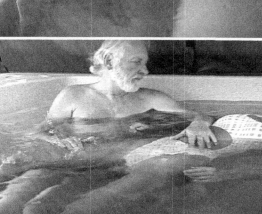

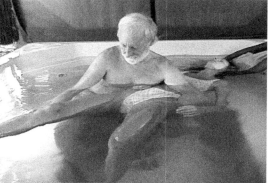

Fourth Post

Picking up the leg, we can move into our fourth post near the feet. Again we can use our legs, this time bracing the back of the knee with one, and the side of the chest with the other, while taking firm hold of the calf we can pull it, creating a powerful full body stretch. While pulling the leg watch the head to make sure it is not pulled off the head cradle, maintaining enough pressure against the side of the chest to keep the head there.

An alternate can be done with the other leg. Instead of bracing the chest with a foot, we can prop the top of the leg over our knee, bracing it against the buttock.

We can work on the calf. The bladder meridian points down its midline are accessible here as well as the spleen meridian points under the shin bone. We can rotate and work on each foot from this third post. We can brace the foot against our body to press and stretch it while working on the points. The major acupuncture point in the bottom of the foot is Kidney 1, a third of the way down from the toes.

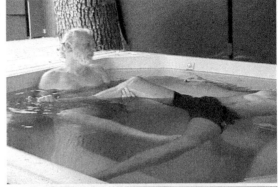

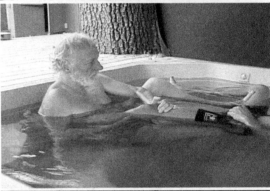

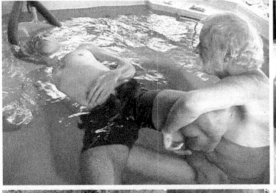

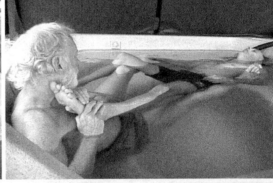

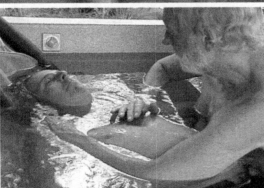

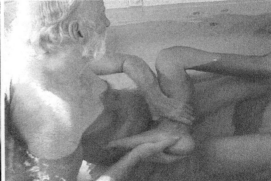

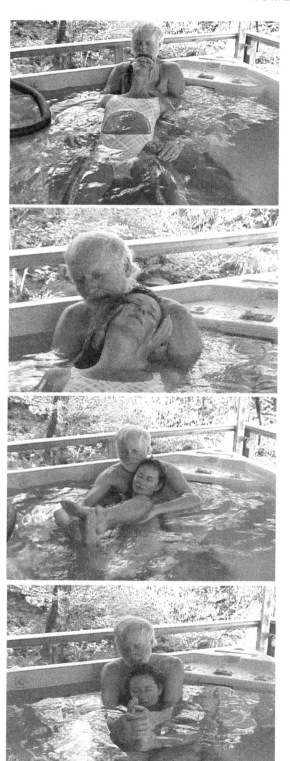

Fifth Post

In the fifth Post we position ourself behind the person. We can bring someone up into a sitting position with their arms still wrapped. This is an excellent position to work on the face and the neck. From this position we can maneuver someone's back against our chest. Avoid hyperextending the neck by not letting the head fall back over your shoulder. If the spa is large enough we can do what is called 'Seaweed', swaying the person from side to side while their head is on our shoulder, and the other moves associated with it in Watsu. We can brace the top of the sacrum with both knees while pulling the head to traction the spine and work the neck. We can rotate both legs, together and alternately.

Second Side

After working on the second foot from the fourth post, if our spa has a bench all the way around we can start back up the second side and, in a reverse order, mirror the work we did in the third, second and first posts. We can leave out some of the moves that have the same effect no matter what side they are done from and add variants such as squeezing the hips from both sides. When we were starting out in the first post on the first side, we maintained support from underneath with one hand while the other worked from above. When we have made our way to the first post on the second side we can more freely explore alternatives such as squeezing the hips from both sides and working into the chest with both hands. We can reach under with both hands and push the elbows together, opening the chest. We can wrap the arms around into a self hug and roll the person.

If you are working in a spa that doesn't have a bench all the way around you can float the person around to work the second side from the same bench. Unless you have prepared a second head cradle, or can easily switch the one to the opposite side, you may be limited to what can be done without laying the head back.

WATSU BASIC AND EXPLORER PATHS

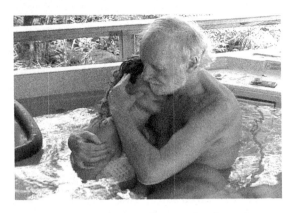

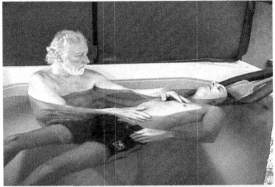

We can catch one foot with the other to bring the feet together and hold them pressed together with the knees splayed outward, stretching the muscles on the inside of the legs. We can suddenly let go in a move we call 'the Spring' in Watsu.

Completion

After such a sudden awakening move, it is good to float someone in stillness, an opportunity for them to integrate within all that has happened.

At the end we return to the position we started from with the hands on the centers, body, heart and mind. Gradually lift both hands off together. Move your legs out from under. Leave them to float in stillness. Wait at their feet.

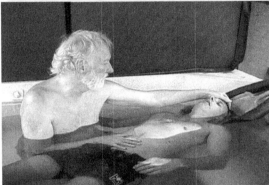

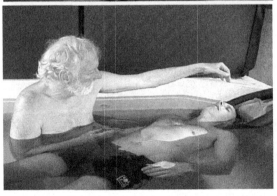

NOTE The above is presented as a progression through the posts and the basic moves we can do at each. Many more stretches and bodywork can be incorporated at each post. Additional work, depending on the size of the spa and its appropriateness can be done from positions kneeling in the water or sitting on the bottom. When you are certain the position would not be misinterpreted, additional work can also be done with someone straddling your lap. In this position you can work down the back, pressing or pulling into the bladder meridian points on each side of the spine. If the spa is large enough to keep the legs straight and at a right angle to the spine, you can also twist stretch someone in this position.

EXPLORATIONS

These explorations of Watsu in words span, in the order they appear, the first twenty years of Watsu's development. Certain basic issues, such as Intimacy, reappear in ever changing form. Down this long hall of mirrors, the farther from the source we go, the closer to the source we come. The concept of oneness, so prevalent at that time, has moved over to make room for wholeness with the work with three.

Nurturing, Bonding, Intimacy and the Oneness Felt During a Watsu

The oneness felt during a Watsu creates a bonding reminiscent of both that between a mother and child, and the bonding between lovers. It creates a space safe enough to experience aspects that had been lacking in earlier bondings, as well as aspects that have been suppressed since painful separations. For many it is the discovery of a level of nurturing they have missed since childhood. It is the discovery of just how much intimacy we can enjoy without any sexual intention underlying it. Discoveries such as these have far reaching effects in a person's life and the quality of 'bonding' they will look for with others. It is imperative that the giver maintain a space within which the receiver can make these discoveries as safe as possible.

For many people the fact they have not been held by anyone in their adult life the way they were held as a child has left a deep craving. Many deny a need exists. In Watsu, as that need is fulfilled, it comes into awareness and can be accepted. The strength and healing the child drew from that source are again available in his or her life. This should not be confused with 'regression.' It is the absence of regression, it is the not having to become a baby to find that source, it is the being able to find that nurturing in the here and now, which gives the experience such power.

The same thing is true of the womb-like experiences many recipients mention. By being moved so freely through the water, by being repeatedly stretched and returned to a fetal position, the adult has the opportunity to heal in himself whatever pain or loss he may still carry from that time. If there is any sense of the restrictions his body grew into within the womb, he may now experience how free his body can be in water. If he has repressed any pain of separation, he can now feel the continuity, the oneness between that time and the present. It is not regression but creation, the power to create in one's own life a wholeness between the past and the present.

Watsu can also help heal wounds to our ability to accept intimacy, whether they were caused through a deprivation of physical contact, or through instances of childhood or later abuse. It can also help people reach a healthier understanding of their own sexuality.

Many problems people have around intimacy are related to their inability (or the people they choose as partners' inability) to distinguish between sexual feeling and sexual intention. Men, in particular, often have this difficulty. They have been trained that a sexual feeling is something to be acted on or repressed. The pressure to act causes them to fantasize a receptivity beyond what might be there. It prevents them from 'being' with another, fully sensitive and attentive to where the other is. In their focus on performance the other becomes an object. The only other way they know how to handle a sexual feeling is to repress it. But repression divides the self, which also makes it difficult to completely 'be' with another.

There are ways of dealing with sexual feeling other than action or repression. This becomes clear during a Watsu where there is no place for sexual intention. In work this close, sexual feelings can come up, but, because there is no way to act on them, they can be enjoyed as pleasurable feelings in themselves, as part of the pleasure the whole body feels being moved continuously through the water. Uncompartamentalized, ungenitalized these feelings can contribute to the release and movement of energy throughout the body, particularly the movement of energy up the spine.

Sexual intention propelled me into bodywork the day I asked a woman sitting beside me in a hot spring pool if she would like a massage (something I had never received in my life let alone given). But the more I worked with bodywork, and particularly with Watsu, the more I felt such connection and joy and fulfillment in the work itself that the imposition of any goal or sexual intention would be out of place. It would be a violation of the trust I felt the person placing in my arms. At the same time I began to feel powerful vibrations of energy rise up my own back, which at the end of a Watsu, would often combine with that of the person I had been working with and rise up over our heads. It was such a bright powerful experience that I began to look for, to anticipate it at the end of each Watsu. But that was substituting another goal, another intention, in place of just 'being' with the person. As I began to let go of that intention, I found that many similar and equally powerful events can occur anyplace during a session when there is no trying to make them happen. It is in this surrender to the moment that we free our bodies, and the more surrendered we become, the more surrendered and freer those we work with become.

Many of those who receive a Watsu speak of feeling their bodies so completely supported and freed that they feel they are flying or sailing through space. Some speak of experiencing cosmic joy or unconditional love, other words for the oneness. My own strongest experience of this occurred this year in a class in Germany where, rather than feeling the rising up my back rise up to join the other's, there was only the one rising up the both of us. The whole pool, and all those around us, were bathed in its light.

Whatever the experience, because it is arrived at through the body's being freed (and not through its being denied), it is an experience that is incorporated in the here and now of the person's life.

There are other intentional modes besides the sexual that should be avoided during a Watsu. Some people may be tempted to play the parent too heavily, not allowing the receiver the freedom to move in and out of whatever state he needs to. Some may distance themselves by holding too close to a doctor/patient model. All such intentions and needs to control fall away as you feel your oneness with the person.

So many people express either verbally, or in their face and body, how much they feel a 'oneness' in (and after) a Watsu that I am convinced that state of 'being at oneness' is crucial to our ability to free our bodies. It provides a context within which our individual limitations are no longer overwhelming. It gives us a new, more accepting perspective on our own and other's lives. In giving the Watsu, the more we feel at one with the other, the freer are our own bodies, and the more individual and unique each session becomes. The more we become one the freer we are to discover our uniqueness. It is as if our uniqueness can only truly unfold in our 'oneness'. And Watsu, at its most creative, becomes a spontaneous celebration of that unfolding.

The water in which we do our Watsu, is itself a symbol of oneness, but when we look a little more closely at water, we see how unique the associations are each person has around it. Water is not the same thing to someone living in a desert as it is to someone who lives by the sea or in a rain forest or in a place threatened by devastating floods.

All of us began our existence in water. Water is the ideal medium for the developing fetus to explore the movement potential in its newly unfolding limbs. Its 'exercise program' begins as early as the eighth week. But being connected as we were to our mothers' emotional states, to her unique rhythms of adrenaline, endomorphine and other hormones and chemicals periodically flooding our common systems, our experiences of womb life are as different as are our mothers.

All of us experienced leaving that watery place, in one way or another. And water has since played so many roles in our lives: what we played and were bathed in, what our wounds were washed in, what many of us were baptized in, what we were warned not to go into by ourselves (especially after eating), what we almost drowned in, what we finally conquered and learned to float and swim in and under and on waves on top of.

To the degree that what water means to us is the sum of all our individual experiences of it, this completely new experience, Watsu, changes what water is. To the degree that our past continues to live in us, this changed meaning reverberates back into and enriches all our memories in which water played a part.

In the same sense Watsu, and the oneness we feel in it, can change in us what it means to be with another; can enrich our understanding of all our relationships.

These changes are gained experientially and not 'intentionally'.

If we intend to change, if we set up a program for ourselves; if we tell ourselves that from this point on we are going to feel unconditional love or oneness with everyone, and then, as inevitably will occur, we feel some judgment or negative feeling toward others, we must suppress that feeling denying a part of ourselves, or feel guilty and inadequate.

With Watsu we feel connections with people that we might never have imagined feeling any connection. No matter what attitude you might have had toward someone, when you feel yourself letting go in their arms, or when, giving a Watsu, you feel someone surrendering, placing such trust in your arms, everything changes.

The more people we feel this unexpected connection with, the more we can free ourselves from the judgments and negative feelings that will still occasionally come up; the more accepting we can be of ourselves knowing how such attitudes dissolve in our 'oneness' in the water.

The Poetics of Watsu

Yesterday Bill Thomson, while interviewing me for an article on Watsu to appear in "East West Journal," pointed out that the group of San Francisco poets I was a member of in the late fifties and sixties were forerunners of today's consciousness raising movements. Exploring correspondences between then and now sheds some light on the origins and nature of Watsu.

I can't imagine anyplace more exciting than San Francisco of the late fifties for a young poet. Besides the almost nightly getting together in the Place in North Beach, and the morning-afters on the lawn at Aquatic Park, there were the regular Sunday meetings where we would read each other our latest poems. I was addicted to writing, and to the state I would get into when a poem would come through on its own; a state I would characterize as one of absolute clarity; of writing with light. Nothing could compare to it. I shunned religion and family and the army and psychoanalysis and anything else I feared might undermine my being a poet (including drugs).

But over the years as the North Beach 'scene' disintegrated in a haze of alcohol, I spent more and more time abroad (two years in Europe, one in Canada and three in Mexico). I no longer had the audience that the Sunday meetings and the White Rabbit and Open Space's publishing of my books provided. I became more and more isolated, an isolation all the more complete because the way I saw myself as a 'poet' set me above the lot of ordinary mortals. I wrote less and less.

When I discovered bodywork I found a way out of that isolation. I found in Watsu, a way to enter with others states similar to what I feel when the poem is coming through most clearly.

I see many correspondences between the poetics that evolved in the late fifties and what happens in Watsu. As poets, freeing the language from its habitual restrictions and limitations was uppermost, just as in Watsu freeing the body is. Both are based on the breath and free rhythms. Both seek places that open us up to possibilities beyond what we can anticipate. Influenced by Zen, both are practices that focus on the here and now, and get us in touch with the unknown. By advocating the kind of freedom they do, both find themselves in opposition to more traditional academic forms; and discover form by breaking through form.

From the beginning I conceptualized Watsu as a sort of poem in motion. I can see my earlier habits of working over and revising poems reappear in the way I work out Watsu sequences for my students. I feel, when Watsu is freest, a creativity at play. This is extremely important in Watsu. There is a need, a drive for creativity in each of us. The more the giver works out of their creativity, the more the receiver feels areas open up that might not have been otherwise accessed. When we move beyond our conscious mind and let go of its need to control, something takes over that knows on a much deeper level just what is needed in the other (who is no longer so much an 'other').

Seeing the origins and effects of Watsu partially embedded in this drive for creativity complements two other aspects of its origin I have already written about: the physical and the emotional (the need for connection with others). Those first two are body and heart, and this third (and the clarity that characterizes it) is mind. Watsu's movement, its dance, frees the body. The closeness and nurturing of Watsu free, and open the heart. And its inventive play and spontaneity free the mind.

In the Boundlessness of Water

Water's strength is in its power to yield, to flow into whatever form would pretend to contain it, to move over and make room for whatever enters it. What better medium could we find in which to learn whatever we need to learn about yielding? In Taoist philosophy this yielding of water is the 'role model' for all our activities, or rather 'non activities' in the world.

The study of the movement of water is the basis of a new science, the science of chaos, which has uncovered a kind of recurrent pattern that seems common to all chaotic events. The freer we get in water, moving with someone, never repeating the exact same movement twice, the more it feels we are moving to a similar kind of 'chaotic' pattern. That pattern might itself facilitate some of the remarkable changes of consciousness experienced during a Watsu. It echoes the chaos that, in so many mythologies, underlies creation and is described as 'the face of the deep', the sea.

Another way water affects our consciousness is what it does to our sense of boundary. This varies dramatically with changes in the temperature of the water. In cold water when the pores of our skin close and the capillaries contract there is a heightened sense of our boundary, and the cold it is trying to keep out from the warmth within. In contrast, when the water is the same temperature as our skin (as it is ideally in Watsu), our pores open and our capillaries dilate, as our body feels more and more boundless.

I am reminded of the five sheaths that surround the atman, the self, in India. Underlying the food sheath, that which we feed and is itself food (for worms and vultures . . . and fire), is the sheath of prana, the warmth, the fire within. Underlying this is the mental sheath, that which sorrows for the body's pain and rejoices in its pleasure. Under this is the wisdom sheath, the innate wisdom of the body. And under this, the sheath of bliss, the rapture that is the foundation of our lives.

The boundlessness felt in warm water is the sheath of prana, the warmth within, becoming one with the warmth of the water. During a Watsu, when our mind's chatter becomes most stilled, the more spontaneous and intuitive our moves become, the more they are coming out of our bodies' innate wisdom, and the deeper we move into rapture.

It is said that once an opening is made to the rapture, once we know how to access it, we will be able to see it underlying even the greatest of our sorrows. I can imagine no better goal for Watsu than to help people realize a level of consciousness from which they can face anything, a level as boundless as water.

Watsu and Continuum

I have just come back from a weekend workshop with Emily Conrad Da'oud, the developer of Continuum. I was impressed with the parallels between what she is doing on land and what we are doing in water. In Continuum emphasis is placed on breaking the 'Neural Lock' that limits our movements to those habitually repeated over and over. Movements outside the habitual provide more neurological information and stimulate the organism. They counter the aging process that accelerates whenever our bodies become locked in habitual patterns. To break those patterns she had us explore both primitive movement and micro-movements. We carry in our bodies the whole history of evolution. When we go into our most primitive movements, the aquatic, we are on our most creative level.

She feels that when we learn and repeatedly practice a set form of movement as with most Yoga and Tai Chi, etc., we are practicing the conclusion of someone else's research, rather than discovering in ourselves those spontaneous movements that express where we are in our own bodies at this moment. Anything less separates us from ourselves. She sees movement that arises out of this deepest level as prayer, as love.

When the watsuer is most deeply connected to his partner, movement does arise out of this level, with a spontaneity and freedom that do not come from either body alone, but from a shared space. The more we watsu from this place, the more neurological information floods both our bodies, and the freer we are to move from within our own bodies when we separate.

I have found over the years that the stretches and meditations I have been doing with my classes have more and more come to incorporate and conclude with getting in touch with the spontaneous movement in the body. How important these Meditation Movements are has become clearer after studying with Emily. I recommend Continuum to anyone interested in Watsu.

Pools I Have Stepped Into

Teaching Watsu, stepping into pools all around the world, I've learned how much you have to adapt and make do with whatever is at hand, whether it's a swimming pool in Montparnasse with fifty watsuers or a hot tub on a boat in Amsterdam. Alongside depth and temperature, a third critical factor is ambience. This is effected by the amount of chlorine in the water, the people around, and the noise and flurry of jets, sprays, and man made currents. I remember one particularly active day at the big spa in Baden Baden where there didn't seem to be any part of the pool not hit by a jet or a spray and my class was stared at with murderous indignation by a family of immigrants from a culture where holding each other must not be OK. Nevertheless the class enjoyed itself that day, and maybe that family did too.

There is no saying what is going on inside someone else's head. One of my students had someone walk up to her while she was giving a Watsu and tell her to stop, that she would frighten children, who, if they saw someone lying so still in her arms, would think he was dead. Another student was told by the management at a spa that his watsuing of a man was disturbing the clientele (watsuing a woman would be OK.) Another time while a Watsu (in bathing suits) was being videotaped, someone went to the manager and complained about the pornographic film being shot in the pool. It is all in the eye of the beholder. There are people who are more threatened and confused by tenderness than by whatever sexual content they can project. We must not allow that to interfere with our ability to give others what we have to give. I've seen many people affected positively by just being around Watsu. Many have told me how calm it made them feel, how just watching put them into a meditative state. Many in the pool spontaneously start to float each other.

Each pool is different. At another spa in Germany we started as a small circle at the relatively quiet center of a big pool. As I demonstrated, a crowd of people began to gather around slowly closing in on us. The next thing I knew they were swinging their arms up over their heads all together, and then straight out to the sides. It was the six o'clock exercise class. We slipped outside.

A more serious pool was one in Austria where I was the only one who could touch bottom. My organizers brought large plastic triangular blocks, but they floated up. They filled them with steel rods, but when someone stood on the blocks they slid around. Straddling two was dangerous. The water had so much chlorine in it everybody's skin was burning. And it was nowhere near warm enough. Finally by the third day it was almost tolerable. But when we came in the next day expecting to find it warm, it was cold. The owner, fearing for the cleanliness of his pool, had added fresh water (and more chlorine) the night before. I will never forget that pool.

But there are many other pools we've been in that are truly unforgettable. I remember the snow covered Alps looming over the huge hot spring pool around the lake from Geneva, steam rising around us. I remember the 22 midwives watsuing each other in a line across the pool outside Venice. I remember the pool in the old people's home in Munich where our last class ended with everybody blissfully floating and drifting together into the corner under a window, the snow falling. Another unforgettable pool is the warm pool in Hawaii, watsuing someone as the ocean's waves break and little fish nibble at our feet. My favorite for classes is the pool Cristina Levi built for Watsu in Tuscany. I've always preferred to teach in a pool at a place that hosts and feeds us, but when I taught in a pool in Madrid where a hundred children with special needs are watsued every week, I felt honored to be in the same water as them.

Stepping Out Of The Pool

The other day in the warm pool someone told me what he found most remarkable in his first Watsu was the way it opened up his chest. He was a massage therapist and had been receiving bodywork for years. He had never had anything affect the intercostals (the muscles between the ribs) the way Watsu did. He pointed out that so much bodywork on land compresses the body whereas Watsu opens it. Besides those actual moves of Watsu that open the chest, and the weightlessness in water, I imagine this effect is enhanced by the way the breath fills the whole body during a Watsu, internally massaging it at the same time the warm water externally massages the body. This opens another line of exploration since the surface of our body, our skin, has in our development originated from the same level as our nerve tissue. It is our brain turned inside out, or rather our brain is our skin turned outside in. Both are being watsued through a sea of feelings and thoughts as broad and limitless as the sea someone steps into when they try to write about something as multidimensional and flowing as Watsu. These explorations could go on forever.

A Separate Path

When I first presented Watsu to the public I was reluctant to call it nonsexual because (1) saying something is not brings up the issue, (2) I didn't want to seem to be against sex, to 'throw out the baby with the bath water' whatever that meant (I have since overcome my inhibitions- Watsu is not sex and the baby is still in the bath water), and (3) they have much in common- the physical intimacy, the heart connection, the ecstatic moments- Both can be paths to the healing inherent in more inclusive states of being. With that in mind, I introduced Watsu as a form of Bodywork Tantra in my book of that title, which was to court misinterpretation in a public which sees Tantra as a form of sex rather than the other way around. If I had been more concerned about what people might think, I would have been more circumspect … and would probably never have developed Watsu. But it is developed, and no one has to repeat whatever mistakes I made while learning how completely separate a path Watsu is. The path is here… and has a potential which can only be realized if its separateness is kept clear. Anyone who fails to do that, who uses Watsu as a tool of seduction, who takes advantage of the trust and openness a Watsu engenders, not only harms the person in their arms. They harm everyone in our Water Family. They harm everyone who might be denied Watsu's benefits because of its being confused with sex.

Besides being aware of and honoring the boundaries of those in our arms, bodyworkers who work in public pools can't help but be aware of how our work might look to the casual observer. The majority of the people who happen on to our work are touched in a very positive way. A few feel threatened. At least two of the many professional writers who have come to write about Watsu have added to this confusion. Writers are observers. Sensitive to what their readers respond to, they observe with the eyes of their public. One writer, a few years back, confused the energy I wrote about in earlier writings with popular conceptions of Tantra and 'sexual energy', as if all the manifestations of energy we experience in our bodies are derived from repressed sexual drives. He observed a woman going into a wavelike ecstasy as I floated her, and identified it with a sexual orgasm. Years later another author referred back to that identification to support her own misgivings about what she felt was Watsu's confusing the boundaries between the sexual and nonsexual. She, too, was there as an observer, observing with the eyes of a public in which women are struggling to become free of sexual exploitation. She wondered how Watsu might be for a victim of sexual abuse. There is no question that, in the hands of someone using Watsu's intimacy and level of trust to fulfill their own sexual agenda, the experience could be devastating. That is why we focus so much on understanding and respecting boundaries in our trainings. Properly and sensitively applied, Watsu can provide those who have been abused a level of healing beyond almost any other approach. In contrast to therapies that focus on the acts of abuse and their effects, Watsu can take people back to what they had before abuse (and still have). It is not uncommon for clients to tell us that this work has done more for them than years of psychotherapy.

Watsu can also reduce the amount of abuse and exploitation there is in the world, by educating people as to how deep a level they can connect on without sexual intention. It can ingrain this knowledge in our beings in a way words alone cannot. One benefit I have received from Watsu, and I see many of the men in our classes receive, is to experience the depth of connection we can have while floating another man in our arms. I have also seen the reactions this can trigger in onlookers. Watsuers have been kicked out of pools for this.

It is important to understand what it is in our work that might seem threatening to an observer. I don't think it is merely a case of projecting repressed sexual feelings and fears. Earlier I mentioned how the need for physical intimacy that we have had since birth is often confused with the need for sex. Our work in water can get people back in touch with that earlier, and separate, need. Some, observing our work, may find it easier to see it as sexual rather than face their own need for unconditional physical intimacy. In a society that sexualizes everything, many repressed needs become confused with the sexual. This may be a way to hide much deeper needs.

All of us have parts of our being whose needs and nature we accept, and other parts we deny or hide. There are some who draw that boundary between their heads and their bodies, who barely tolerate any needs that their bodies might have. These, who are in the greatest need, are not likely to turn up on a massage table or in our pools. Being touched by a barber or a doctor may be the only form of touch they accept outside of their immediate family.

Others draw the boundary between being touched and being held. To those who deny any need to be held, shaking hands is OK but hugging is not. There is a qualitative difference between being touched and being held. This can be seen by imagining the deprivation of an infant who is touched but never picked up and held, a mother's instinctive way of healing a child in pain.

Watsu is a holding therapy. It allows people to experience being held in a way that is completely natural, in a medium, water, in which being held is necessary, and which itself holds them.

Another area where people may create a boundary is between the head and the heart (or the heart and the body). The degree to which the heart has its own mind is being documented through research at the Institute of HeartMath in Boulder Creek. They have found that many emotional states show up in the heart's electromagnetic field before they appear in the brain. They have also found profound effects occur when there is entrainment between the heart's rhythms and other rhythms such as that of the breath. In Watsu, when we have connected our breathing and are floating someone level with our heart, there is a powerful sense of heart connection. The receiver typically feels a great sense of peace. The entrainment throughout the body and the resonance between the chakras will occasionally, in a body floating freely, show up as an ecstatic wavelike or vibratory movement which may fulfill another need not always recognized- that of feeling the freedom of our body and its energy, which may have an even deeper need underlying it, that of reconnecting to our source.

At the Heart of Watsu

I continue to be amazed at the connection we feel when we coordinate our breathing and float someone level with our heart center. Research at the Institute of HeartMath (www.heartmath.com) sheds light on what I've called a 'heart wrap' ever since I began developing Watsu twenty five years ago.

Listening in on the heart, and tracking its effects, researchers confirm what traditional cultures take for granted. The heart has a mind. Its forty thousand neurons store information and make decisions. Through nerves, pulse, hormones and an electromagnetic field four thousand times stronger, the heart communicates with the brain, and every part of the body.

When someone feels the kinds of feelings often felt during a Watsu- care … appreciation … love … the variability in the Heart's rhythms show up as regularly recurring waves. The heart is the body's strongest oscillator. The same waves show up in the brain, respiration, and other systems. This coherence allows the heart to fulfill its role as the manager of our emotions. Entrained to the heart, the brain can focus on areas where its more analytical intelligence is needed. Our overall creativity is enhanced.

Those at HeartMath also find that under stress these waves become chaotic and disconnected. When we experience (or recall) anger the chaotic rhythms continue for many hours afterwards. In this chaotic state our immune system is weakened and our sympathetic, fight or flight, nervous system over-activated. The perpetuation of this state, and the increasing difficulty to return to coherence, underlies most of our modern illnesses.

The nurturing holding and gentle movement of Watsu can bring both giver and receiver into heart coherence. I have always felt that the connection that comes with our 'heart wrap' is a connection to everything, a oneness, a level of being from which we can look with equanimity on what would otherwise disturb us. I realize now that that is heart coherence. If the person in our arms is in their own coherence, it may be a unique opportunity for them to let whatever they have been suppressing, or obsessing on, with the emotionally incompetent brain, find a place in the heart's understanding. In Watsu we call this 'letting things go into the flow'. We never interrupt a Watsu to ask what is wrong when we see tears come to someone's eyes. At the end of a session, we never pry for details. Asking someone to recall events behind whatever came up may throw them back into the chaotic state that Watsu has been leading them away from, and undo Watsu's most valuable gift. Watsu is at the opposite pole from therapies that posit reliving past traumas or catharsis as the way to release them, something that those at HeartMath also find counterproductive.

Since both giving and receiving Watsu enhances one's ability to move into coherence, the next step to further the healing received from Watsu is to share it with others. I realize now that the 'presence' we look for in our Watsu students is heart coherence. Our earlier trainings burdened our students with too much material. The stress of learning so much kept them in a chaotic state that made it difficult to develop presence. A few years ago this changed when I introduced the Water Breath Dance. Its breath connected heart wrap in which giver and receiver surrender together to the water helps students develop presence from the beginning. This move (or non-move), and the way we come 'home' to it throughout a session, distinguishes Watsu from other forms of water work. It brings into reach our goal of making the benefits of both giving and receiving the simple forms of Watsu available to everybody.

The HeartMath findings show us why we have taken the direction we have and point to the work that lies ahead- helping people access and stay longer in their coherence in and out of the water. For some the way on land may be recalling being watsued, letting everything go into that flow. Those who experienced giving Watsu may return to that state by watsuing others in their heart-mind. The author, Alma Flor, once told us how she 'watsued' her academic colleagues as they argued around a table ... and whole audiences as she lectured to them. If, as they say at HeartMath, not being able to forgive someone can keep us from coherence, what better partners could we have in our arms than those we most need to forgive? Imagine a city in which everybody walks down the street lovingly watsuing each other.

The way I find to return to the coherence of Watsu on land is to sink into the emptiness that we sink into at the bottom of the breath in the Water Breath Dance. In HeartMath I finally find an explanation for the wave that vibrates my body when I sink deepest into that emptiness. It is the body's entrainment to the heart's coherent rhythm. Because I often feel it initiated at the level of the heart when I embrace a friend and 'listen' to his or her heart with my heart, I've been calling it a heart-bodywave. We occasionally see this wave in someone when, after strong stretches and moves, we bring him or her home to the stillness of the Water Breath Dance. It was my own experience of this the first time someone floated me at Harbin Hot Springs, and wanting to share it with others, that started me developing Watsu, incorporating the stretches and moves of the Zen Shiatsu that I practiced and taught there.

Our waves resonate with those we float. At HeartMath they record the change of rhythms in people touching and find resonances that point to some kind of shared coherence (a coherence I feel as rising to, resonating with, everything). I feel that bringing us back to that oneness is how the heart mind manages our emotions. Another area of research finds that as meditators approach their most powerful experiences of oneness, changes are measured in that part of the brain that otherwise tracks their position in space and maintains their sense of physical boundary. The boundlessness of Water, and the disorientation being moved in it with eyes closed, all add to the oneness in a Watsu. And Oneness is the only place from which everything can be let go. And the more that is let go the emptier is the Emptiness, the place that is the source of all our creativity, of all healing, of every wave.

Research makes it clearer what is at the heart of Watsu. My heart mind feels understood. We can all have a little more clarity about the waves our love is making in the world.

Birthright

Breath is life
The body is movement
And the base of our being
Is the support of others

WOGA

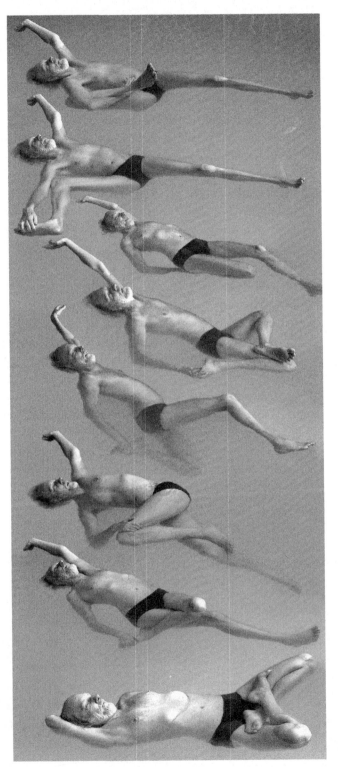

Water is ideal for stretching, for Water Yoga. Depending on the available depths, this can be done standing, sitting and lying, as well as floating. If there is a bar, many stretches can be improvised at the wall. What follows is a sequence that can be done while floating in the state of tonus described in the previous section. Besides opening up those parts of the body being stretched, doing this while floating provides opportunities to explore extension in parts not being held in a stretch.

Leg Wrap

Float on your back, your arms up over your head. Move your right knee as near to the right side of your chest as possible. Hook your right elbow under it and place your right hand on your hara just below the navel. Float.

Pull Wide

Remove your right hand from your hara and hold your right foot, pulling your right leg straight. Feel how wide out your left arm and leg spread as you stretch the muscle down the back of your right leg.

Heel Up

Hold your right foot near the toes and press the heel of your right foot into your right buttock. Hold and feel the powerful straight line of extension up left arm and down left leg.

Flying W

Press your right foot up to the surface, lifting with your right hand under the inside of your right foot. Prop your left foot over your right thigh. Let your left arm curve up over your head. Float.

Pull Under

Slip your left foot off your right thigh as you reach under with your right hand and pull the left foot towards your right side. Let the rest of your body reach out in whatever way balances and amplifies this stretch.

Twist

Release the left foot. With your right hand pull your left knee across the top of your right thigh to twist stretch your spine.

Leg Over

Pull your left foot towards the side of your right hip, wrapping your left knee around your right thigh.

Lotus

If you are comfortable in lotus position, slide your left ankle over the top of your right leg. Reach down with your right hand and prop the other ankle over the top of the other leg. Float and explore movement in lotus. If you can hook your fingers behind your back, one arm under your head and the other under your waist, you will find yourself tied up in a way that supports your head and allows you to float freely.

Second Side

Float with your arms up over your head and repeat the mirror image of the above on the second side.

Knees Up

Wrap your upper arms (coming from between) around your knees to press them to your chest.

Feet pull

Hold your feet, the bottoms pressed together, with both hands and float.

Both Heels Up

Holding a foot in each hand, press their heels up towards your buttocks and float.

Shake Free

Straighten your legs and float, allowing vibration or shaking to work its way up your body in stronger and stronger waves. Notice how those waves' changing as they pass up your head and neck can lead you into a state of total ecstasy, how everything around you becomes brighter, and freer. As the undulations coming up your spine become stronger and stronger, be careful to not let your head jerk back so violently it strains your neck. If that becomes a danger, try accessing the same waves while standing (or kneeling) under water where your spine is vertical and your head has the support of the water.

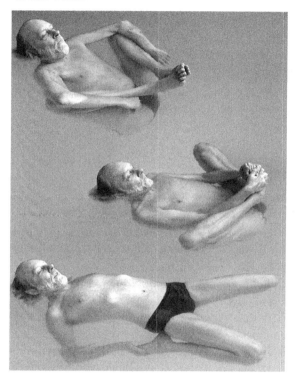

WATSU BASIC AND EXPLORER PATHS
CREATIVE MOVEMENT MEDITATIONS

Creative movement is the movement that arises spontaneously when we are most present in our body, when our body is most free. Because it is creative, there is no limit to the forms it can take. Its most basic form is that of the wave. Creative movement is internally generated. It comes from within and spreads freely through the body. It may or may not be externally visible. On the cellular level it is continuous. Its presence defines life. It can be manifested in swift vibrations rising up the spine, or in very slow undulations of our body. Emptying into the void at the bottom of the breath, getting in touch with the flows of our meridians, and connecting our chakras are ways to open ourselves up to creative movement. Water is ideal. It allows a greater amplitude of wave motion than being on land. Our bodies are made of water and they still have within them memories of all the forms of water experienced in our personal development and in the evolution of life. These can be accessed on land. The following opens with movement in water and then moves on to three Movement Meditations on land. If you are not in a pool, skip ahead to the meditations on land.

THE WATER WAY

The following presents ways you can explore the connection and freedom of your body in water. As with Watsu, the ideal place for exploring these comfortably and slowly, is in water the temperature of your body's surface. If the water is cooler, you may need to intersperse moments of faster, more active movement.

The Waterbreath Dance

There is a simple practice you can do in a pool to coordinate your breathing with your body's letting go in the water. Settle into water that is two thirds as deep as your height, your legs spread as wide as is comfortable, each foot staying in its place, your arms floating out in front of you. As you breathe out let your body sink straight down (keeping your nose out). Feel how, as you breathe in, the water lifts you back up, and how, as you breathe out, it lets you back down. Notice any holding in your knees or elsewhere. When you breathe out, sinking, let go of it a little more. Surrender to the water. At the bottom of the breath, is a moment of total stillness, of emptiness, before the breath and the water start you back up. Keep doing this until you feel one with your breath and the sinking and rising, until you feel it is the water breathing you up and down, until you feel one with the water, your partner, in this Waterbreath Dance.

Sinking

To be completely comfortable in water both sinking and floating should be as natural to you as your own breath. To explore sinking on a deeper level take three deep breaths and, blowing all the air out, let yourself settle to the bottom. Lying on your back do a series of swift abdominal contractions and then lie perfectly still. Feel how comfortable it is to lie on the bottom, and how long you can lie without breath (Don't try this in a crowded pool ... nor in a completely empty pool ... Have someone around in case you forget to come up). When you do come back up, do it slowly without rushing or panic, and, when your head comes out of the water don't gasp for air but breathe in naturally. Learning to lie on the bottom of a pool without fear may have further benefits. I remember the sense of empowerment the first time I lay quietly at the bottom not unlike what someone must feel after fire walking.

Tai Chi in Water

Water is ideal for slow, Tai-chi like movement. Our basic Water Dance, and the Watsu itself, is done in this spirit. Alone in the pool, as you sink into the Water Dance, let your body settle into and come back up out of the water. Each time your head goes under, let the completion of your body's movement bring your head back out rather than the desire to breathe, or the fear of running out of breath. When you do come up, take your time and breathe in slowly. See how completely your body's movements can be coordinated with your breathing without intention or fear. Explore how every movement leads to its completion and opens to another movement. Explore all the connections of movement.

Floating

The more body fat you have, the easier it is to float. Even those with a limited amount of fat can learn to float, if they practice controlling their breath and the tonus of their body. A way of breathing that can help you float is to always maintain a reservoir of air in your lungs by never completely emptying them. The tonus can be achieved by keeping your arms stretched up over your head and your legs straight, at the same time as you keep your whole body relaxed.

Three States

Have someone stand beside you, one hand under the back of your head, the other under your sacrum while you lie back in the water, your arms straight up over your head. Imagine your whole body is as rigid as steel. Tighten every muscle in your body. Feel how heavy you are in the water. Next imagine your whole body is rubber, totally limp. Feel how your body would sink if someone wasn't holding you. Now imagine your whole body is wood, not the wood in a piece of furniture but the wood in a living tree. Feel the life of a tree from the tips of your toes all the way up to your fingertips. Feel the resiliency of wood, how different it is than the stiffness of steel and the limpness of rubber. Feel how much easier it is to float when you feel this extension of life throughout your body. At this point the person holding you can move down to below your feet and gradually remove support from under them.

A Smile on the Face of the Deep

Water is in our every cell. We know it in all its shapes and forms. In water explore whatever way that body or form of water allows. Outside explore all the forms and movements of water that our body comes to know, wave, river, undertow, water spout, still pond. Water is shape changing. And so are our bodies. All the states and forms from our individual development, from the evolution of life, and from creation itself when everything appeared in the Face of the Deep. Where we can most feel this in our own bodies is in the emptiness at the bottom of the breath, when, rather than following the breath out, we center in the emptiness left behind. This is the moment in the breath cycle when our diaphragm and our abdominal muscles have most completely relaxed, the moment before they become activated again as we breathe in. If we center and ground ourselves in this emptiness, there is no part of creation that we cannot experience rising up out of it, and returning back into it. The way of the breath, the way our bodies move to it, the way we empty into the void at the bottom of the breath, and are raised back up out of it in waves, is the focus of the first Movement Meditation. In the second we stretch our meridians and focus on the energy pathways in our body in a way that take us through another cycle of creation. A third creation cycle is experienced in the last meditation when we connect our centers or chakras. The three Movement Meditations can be each practiced separately, or as one long uninterrupted process. The more we experience creation, and its flows and centers, within our bodies, the more we will find our bodies opening to spontaneous creative movement. Feel free to spend as long as needed when this starts to happen. These meditations are as flexible and adaptable to individual needs as the bodywork in this book. If you are following this on video or audio cassette, have a pause button near at hand and use it whenever you are in a place where you feel the opportunity to further explore movement (or stillness).

When doing the following it is best to be in a room with a rug comfortable enough to lie on. Wear clothing loose enough to stretch in. When asked to sit, sit in whatever position is comfortable and best helps keep your back straight. If you are going to need a cushion, or a chair, have one near by.

BREATH AND WAVE

In the following you will stand, rocking your body to your breath, and explore how your breath and body become one. You will get down on hands and knees and explore how your body opens to the filling and emptying of the breath. You will sit and enter even deeper into that emptiness at the bottom of the breath, which is the void before creation (The Face of the Deep). You will explore the wave movement in your own body, which is the movement of life rising out of that void. You will explore the aquatic, the animal and the human dance. You will stand and hold in your hands the peace that is at the center. You will lie in the wave.

The Way of the Breath Rocking

Stand, legs spread as wide as is comfortable, shoulders relaxed, arms hanging loose to your sides, face and neck relaxed, hips and knees. Breathe out slowly, slowly settling into your body, your knees bending. Breathe in slowly straightening your legs. Feel how your body rises up as the breath fills it. Each time you breathe out let your body sink to whatever direction, and as deeply, as it wants. Each time you breathe in feel that rising up your spine, all the way up your body. Explore all the ways your body might want to sink as it lets go into the outbreath, as your breath empties and your body empties with it. Enjoy the sinking into that emptiness, and the rising up out of it each time you breathe. Your body is one with your breath. Gradually build up the pace of your breathing. Breathe faster and faster. Your body, rocking to your breath, sinks and rises faster and faster. Your arms start swinging by themselves to its rocking. Let them swing to whatever direction and as high as they want. Notice how it is your breathing that is rocking and swinging your body and arms. When it has reached a joyful, playful pace, when it is dancing free to your breath, gradually slow down your breathing. Slower and slower, your body rocking slower and slower. Slow it down until the rocking becomes totally internal, until your body is no longer visibly moving. Feel how there is still an internal sinking each time you breathe out, and a filling, a rising each time you breathe in. Feel how even in stillness there is an internal rocking, a sweet pulsing of the breath. Breath and body are one. *(Pause)*

The Way of the Breath Opening

Slowly get down on your hands and knees, spreading them as wide as is comfortable. Keeping your shoulders relaxed, and your arms straight, slowly rock forward as you breathe out, and back as you breathe in, but not so far back that any effort is required to rock forward again. Keep your neck relaxed. Each time you rock forward, feel the letting go in your center just below your navel. Each time you breathe in and rock back feel the rising up your spine. Continue rocking to the breath this way until it becomes totally automatic, until breath and body are one. Sit as far back between your knees as is comfortable. Place your elbows on the floor in front of your knees, your head dropped between them. Without moving externally, continue to feel the breath rising up your spine and emptying back into your center. Stay as open to this breath as a hollow tube. Feel how at the very bottom of the breath, there is an emptying all the way into the perineum, and how, from that point between your legs, there is a rising all the way up your spine as you breathe in. Enjoy the peace that comes with being open, with being one with the emptying and filling that breathes in the stillness. *(Pause)*

The Way of the Breath Emptying

Sit in whatever position best helps keep your back straight and is comfortable. If necessary, place a cushion under your tailbone, or sit on the edge of a chair. Rest your hands, palms up, in your lap, one hand lying in the other, the tips of your thumbs touching. Relax face, neck, shoulders, back, sacrum, buttocks and the rest of your body. Feel how straight your spine can be without effort. Feel how as you breathe in, the filling rising up your spine, is a wave spreading out to all parts of your body. And how, as you breathe out, all those parts settle and empty into the center. Be aware of any part that doesn't empty as much as the rest and, the next time you breathe in, fill that part even more. As you breathe out, let it, let everything empty into the center.

Be aware of the whole area around the center, the navel— the front, the sacrum— the back, and the perineum— the bottom. This whole area around the center is a bowl at the base of the spine. Each-time you breathe out, everything empties into that bowl ... and rises up out of it each time you breathe in. At the very bottom of the breath when everything has emptied into that bowl, for a moment, the bowl itself is empty. When everything has emptied into that bowl, the bowl empties into that point at the bottom, the first chakra. This is where our energy returns into the void, which is its most powerful state, because it is pure potential. At the bottom of each breath empty into that void. Notice what happens as the breath starts up your body again. Let whatever opens to it, open. Let whatever moves to it, move. Movement is life. And out of that stillness in the void comes all life. There is no part of your being that is not at this moment moving out of that stillness. Every bone, every muscle, every cell is moving, however slightly, wave upon wave. You are the Face of the Deep. Smile. *(Pause)*

The Way of the Wave

Every movement begins as a wave. Begin the waves that are your arms and legs, and get down on all fours, on hands and knees, a wave rocking your body into whatever shape it wants, rocking you back and forth. The waves bring you up onto your hands and knees and rock you, wave upon wave. Your spine, flexible, moves to whatever waves rise up out of the void and wash you up onto the shore. And that void continues to flow into whatever shape it rocks your body, into whatever animal crawls up out of that void, into whatever growl or laugh comes out of your throat. There is nothing that does not come out of the void, wave upon wave. *(Pause)*

When the void has completed its crawling up over the earth, let the wave lift you up to stand. Stand. Hold the area around your center, around your navel, in both hands. From the animal comes the human, human hands holding human center, human spine upright, but still flexible, still wavering in the waves that rise up. Feel the peace in your hands. Hold it in your hands as the waves rise through your body. Feel that peace in your center as the waves slowly move your arms out in front of you, as the waves rock and move your whole body, freer and freer, your spine moving, turning, spiraling in whatever waves rise up it. Everything is moving in waves. And however freely arms, legs, neck, head move there is still a unity, a oneness, a joy in the dance, a stillness. That peace is as much one with all these waves as is the particle in the waves of matter. Focus on the stillness in each wave as your arms lower, as your body's movement slows down and becomes still. Feel the inside of the waves, the hollow places under the waves, moving without movement in your body. Still. Stand still. Still dance. Still.

Slowly lower yourself to the floor and lie back, your arms spread out to the sides. Settle into the floor as into the waters of a warm ocean, its slow gentle waves slowly rocking your body in waves. There is no difference between whatever waves you feel within your body and whatever waves slowly lift and rock your body. They are all one wave. Your body and your breath and your rock are all one wave that goes on and on and on. There is no end to the wave.

MERIDIANS STREAMING

In the following you will stretch the meridians of the legs and explore how they connect us to the earth and the power we get from and return to the earth. You will stretch the meridians of the arms and explore how they open to the outside and protect the inside. You will get in touch with other energy pathways, our breathing and our senses, and how they also have a yin and a yang flow.

Opening our Connections to the Earth

Stand, facing the center of the room, knees slightly bent. The breath pulses. It is oceanic. Movement from within goes out through the body in waves. Meridians are steady flows along the surface of the body. Stand still. Focus on the surface. One pair, the central meridians, flows up the back and down the front. It is a lake the other meridians flow out of as rivers, each bearing its share of our life force, their functions related to where they flow. There is a flow all the way down the front of your body. The meridian of the front begins just under the eyes and flows down chest, belly, legs, all the way down. We go out in front of ourselves to get food, our sustenance from the earth. There is a flow all the way down the sides of your body. The meridians of the side begin to the outside of the eyes and flow down both sides down shoulders, hips, ankles, all the way down. They have to do with deciding which way to go, this way or that, with our power, with how we use the energy we get from the earth. There is a flow all the way down the back. The meridian of the back begins to the inside of the eyes and flows up over the top of the head and all the way down the back, water flowing down the back, down the back of the legs. It has to do with elimination, with purification, with what we leave behind and return to the earth, or don't, and still carry on our back.

All these meridians that start around the eyes, that flow down front, sides and back, flow down to the earth. Follow that flow down to the earth, all the way down. Get down on the earth. Get down on your knees and lean back, placing your hands on the earth behind you. Keep your arms straight. Keep hands and knees grounded, planted in the earth. Raise your hips higher and higher. Stretch the meridian of the front, the meridian of the earth. Arch it up as curved as the earth. Hold it as long, and stretched as high, as you comfortably can.

Lower your hips and slide your legs out from under. Straighten and spread your legs out to the sides as wide as possible. Raise your hands up in the air. To stretch the meridian of decision and power, decide what side you're going to stretch toward. Decide and, keeping your chest facing forward and open, lean to that side. Feel the power opening, stretching the side you are leaning away from. Each time you breathe out feel the stretch open up more. Straighten up and lean to the other side. What you feel being stretched is the meridian of the green that grows out of the earth.

Straighten, arms still up over your head. Bring your legs closer together, straightened out in front of you. Keep your back and arms and legs straight. Slowly swing forward to stretch the meridian of the back. Feel its stretch all the way down the back of your legs. This is the meridian of water. If we could let go of all that we carry, our backs would be water. On each outbreath sink a little deeper into the stretch. Do not rock but stay as you breathe in, and sink a little deeper as you breathe out, feeling it slowly open to its flow.

Slowly lower yourself back on the floor, arms out to the sides. Lie still and feel whatever flows these stretches have opened up in your body. *(Pause)* When you feel the flow down the front of your body, feel the earth in your body lying on the earth and its movements. When you feel the flow down the back, feel the water your body is spreading out over the earth, and its movement. When you feel the flows down the sides, feel the richness of new life watered and growing out of the earth, and its movement.

Grow out of the Earth. Slowly raise your knees and pull them to your chest. Hugging them to you with both arms, feel the roundness of the earth in your body. Lay your right arm out to the right, and keep your right shoulder on the ground, as you slowly lower your bent knees to your left and twist over the earth as slow as a vine. Pull your knees back up and hold them to you again. Lay your left arm out and slowly twist to your right. Continue rolling to the right until you roll up onto your knees, spreading them as wide as is comfortable. Rest your forehead on the earth. Keep your hands rooted in the earth you grow out of, as you straighten your arms, and raise your knees off the ground, your feet spread and rooted in the earth. Slowly walk your hands towards your feet as your legs straighten up, your waist still bending over the earth you grow out.

Inside and Outside

Each one of the three Yang meridians, whose flow you followed down the outside of your body, has a Yin partner that flows up the inner surfaces of your legs. Feel that flow up from the earth your legs are still rooted in. Keep your arms hanging toward the earth and slowly straighten your back vertebra by vertebra. Follow that yin flow up the inside of the legs, up through the hara, up to the area around the heart. This is the area where all the yin flows up the arms begin. When your back is straight let that rising Yin slowly raise your arms up in front of you. Feel that flow of Yin up their inner surfaces. When your arms are raised as high as the highest branches of a tree, reach up into the Yang and feel its flow down the outside of your arms. Each of the three Yin meridians in the arm has a yang partner that flows down the outside, down into neck and face where all the Yang meridians that flow down the legs begin. The Yang flow from Heaven to Earth, down the outside. The Yin flow from Earth to Heaven, up the inside.

Spread your arms out at an angle midway between straight up and straight out, the angle which best opens your chest. Stretch them back to open the chest more and more. What is stretching now is the pair of meridians that have to do with the interchange between the inside and the outside. This is the stretch that opens this pair to the outside. Feel how open your lungs are. To stretch the same meridians to the inside, lower your arms and hook your thumbs behind your back. Pull your shoulders back. As you breathe out, bend forward at the waist and swing your arms, thumbs still hooked, vertical up over your back. Hold. Stretch the arms further forward each time you breathe out. Come up slowly and stand still a moment, letting your arms hang at your side. Feel the openness between the inside and the outside.

There is a deeper inside. Raise and bend your right arm behind your head. Hold your right elbow with your left hand and pull it toward your left shoulder. This stretches the meridians that have to do with that deepest inside— the heart. It opens them to the outside. Change arms behind your head and stretch your left arm toward your right shoulder, opening that side to the outside. To stretch the same meridians to the inside, lower your arms and, facing the center of the room, sit on the floor. Hold your feet in your hands and pull them into you as close as possible, the soles of your feet pressed together, your knees spread out and as close to the floor as possible. Surrender the straightness of your back. Round it forward, stretching your whole being around your inside, around that deepest center in your chest.

Sit up and cross your legs. Sit in whatever position best helps you keep your back straight. Raise your arms straight up, palms forward. Swing them back to stretch up their midline. The meridians you are stretching open to the outside now are the ones that have to do with the surface, with what protects that deepest center we stretched around before, and what comes to the surface from that center. To stretch the same to the inside, keep your back straight, cross your arms and pull your opposite knees without swinging them up.

Pathways All Around

Rest your hands on your lap, one in the other, palms up, thumbs touching. Sit, your back straight. Focus on the meridians' flows in your body. You have stretched the meridians in your legs that connect you to the earth and its power, and those in your arms that open to

the outside and protect the inside. There are other energy pathways. Our senses reach out way beyond our arms. Our senses are energy pathways that also come in yin and yang pairs. With eyes closed focus on sight. Looking is yang. It is a going out, and seeing is yin. It is an accepting in. Behind closed eyelids, look. See. Listening is Yang, and hearing Yin. Listen. Hear. Touch is Yang, and feeling Yin. Without moving touch the space around your hands, the clothes around your body. Feel that space and the clothes on your skin. So much of the time we look without seeing, we listen without hearing, we touch without feeling. See. Hear. Feel. And the breath is an energy pathway. What rises as we breathe in is Yang, and what empties as we breathe out is Yin. Open up to the Yin at the bottom of the breath. Completely empty into that emptiness. It is our grounding place within. The more we ground in it the freer flow the central meridians, those that rise up the back and settle down the front, that lake that all the others flow out of. Still water.

CENTERS RESONATING

In the following you will explore how your energy centers can be connected in ways that recreate the creation cycle outlined in the Taoist canon, the Tao Te Ching. You will explore the ways your body spontaneously moves to the resonances established between the centers at each stage of creation. You will explore creation and how at the bottom of every breath we return to the moment before.

The Tao And The One Being Born

Sit, hands in your lap, thumbs touching, a circle. As you breathe in feel the rising up your back, a wave spreading out to all parts of your body. As you breathe out feel how all those parts let go and settle and empty into the center. Be aware of the whole area around the center, the navel — the front, the sacrum — the back, and the perineum — the bottom. It is a bowl at the base of the spine. Each time you breathe out, everything empties into that bowl. At the very bottom of the breath, when everything has emptied into that bowl, the bowl itself empties into the point at the bottom, the first chakra, which is where our energy returns into the void, which is its most powerful state because it is pure potential. In the *Tao Te Ching* Lao Tzu says,

> The Tao gives birth to the One
> The One gives birth to the Two
> The Two gives birth to the Three
> And the Three to the Ten Thousand

What you feel in that void at the bottom of the breath is the Tao, the undifferentiated, the mother of all beings. What you feel rising up your back as you breathe in is the Tao giving birth to the One. The One is your crown chakra, where you are one with everything. Empty into that void, into the Tao at the bottom of the breath, and feel how, as you breathe in, the One is being born all the way up your back, all the way up the back of your head, all the way up to that place of light, not a seeing light but a being light, a shining out to all sides. And as you breathe out, feel how all that light settles back down the front, as slow as snow falling, darkening as it empties back into the Tao.

The Deepest Heart Center

We have been using our breath as a vehicle, but this rising up the back and settling down the front is a continuous cycle. And the Tao is continuous. And the One is continuous. Where we can most feel its continuity is midway between the rising and the settling, midway between the Tao and the One, at the center of that whole continuous circle, in the deepest center in the heart center.

As you focus on this deepest center be aware of what your body is doing, or wants to do. This is our most personal, most private, most vulnerable center. Our bodies develop ways to protect it. Feel how your body protects it, maybe a tightening, a drawing in of your shoulders. Let it. But the next time you breathe out let all that protection and vulnerability and pain settle and empty back into the Tao. As you breathe in feel how open your heart center can be. Feel that openness in your arms. Slowly raise them and hold them out in front of you, a circle, your fingers almost touching, palms facing your heart center. Feel the openness of your heart center in your arms, arms that hold those you love. Let those arms and your torso freely dance that loving openness. *(Pause)* When it has fully opened, lay your two hands, one on top of the other, over your heart center, still holding its openness.

The Two

Lay your hands on your knees, palms up. Just as there is a deep center in your heart, there is a deep center in your mind. Focus on these two at the same time. As you focus on these two, notice whatever movement, or tendency to move, there is in your body. Maybe a rocking from side to side, or a spiraling. As it moves so, notice how these two never come any closer together, and never move any further apart, but dance, forever maintaining the same distance. These are the Two that are born out of the One- Heart and Mind, Soul and Spirit, Yin and Yang. These are the two poles of all the meridian pairs that create and maintain the life of your body. Feel the wholeness of their flow from head to feet to heart, and from heart to hands to head. Feel what a beautiful creation your body is, a creation of the dance of Heart and Mind.

The Three

The body has its own center on the surface, just below the navel. And the Heart has a center on the surface, the Heart Chakra. And the Mind has a center on the surface, the Third Eye. These are the three you face the world with, your strength, your love, your clarity. As you focus on these three notice whatever movement your body begins to make. Maybe a rocking forward this time because these are the three you face the world with. Notice how these three resonate together. It is not pulse nor flow but resonance that connects our chakras. But they are not always in harmony, in balance. Notice whatever balance there is between these three now.

The Ten Thousand

Midway between the body center and the heart center, in the solar plexus, is the center of your will, of your actions, of your deeds. Your deeds realize the balance, or the lack of it, between your body's strength and your heart's love. Midway between the heart chakra and the third eye is the center in your throat, the center of your communications, of your words. Your words realize the balance, or the lack of it, between your heart's love and your mind's clarity. Your words and your deeds are the Ten Thousand that are born out of the three. All Ten Thousand, everything you have ever said or done, everything you are still proud of for the balance it has shown, or are still ashamed of for its lack, all Ten Thousand are a wall in front of you. However tall, however wide that wall, the next time you breathe out let it all slowly crumble and fall. Let all you have ever said or done settle and empty back into the Tao. As you breathe in, feel how balanced the Three can be. Let the Three settle and empty back into the Tao. And the Two and their dance. Let the Two dance their way back into the Tao. And the One, and all that light. Let everything settle and empty back into the Tao.

The Right Person in the Right Place at the Right Time

The Right Place
Harbin Hot Springs

In the more than forty countries I have been to, I have never found, or heard, of anyplace as free, as open, and as ideal for the development of Watsu as Harbin Hot Springs. It is not an ashram. There is no guru or cult leader heading it, no doctrine. When Robert Hartley bought its 5000 acres and run down buildings in 1972, he invited people to move in and help re-build and manage it. When I arrived about 150 were in the community. There were three or four places where workshops were held. It was clothing optional (our Watsu classes were not). Thousands of visitors came every week from the San Francisco Bay Area and around the world. We had our own center for Watsu for the five most important years in the development of Watsu. I taught at Harbin every year until it was destroyed in one of California's biggest wildfires in 2015.

The Right Time

1980 was at the height of the Sexual Revolution, an age of exploration. Aids had not yet appeared. Silence had not yet been decreed for Harbin's warm pool and we could discuss the new moves we enjoyed trying out in it. I moved into a little building near the pools where I offered Zen Shiatsu. The next year someone brought a massage school to Harbin. I bought the School and added a Watsu practitioner certification program the last year it would have been possible. The next year, in order to stop vocational schools from getting government grants for trainings in fields with few employment opportunities, the state passed a law that in order to keep a program, a school had to prove 70 % of its graduates were employed full time in that field. We created and sold the school to a non-profit, the only exemption from this requirement (and even a non-profit could not add a Watsu program without commitments from future employers). The non-profit, WABA, served also to get Watsu around the world. If we had not been able to integrate Watsu into our school and encourage our massage students to attend it, it is impossible to say how far and how soon Watsu would spread.

The Right Person

Fools rush in where angels fear to tread.

My many years practice of Tantra prepared me to walk up in the pool to a naked woman that I had never met before and offer to float her, knowing that the trust with which she lies back in my arms is something that I could never violate. All women and men are beautiful when they surrender into our arms whether they are naked or not. It is a beauty we see and feel without looking. A greater sense of boundaries would prevent most people from starting Watsu this way, particularly boundaries that they carry within to prevent themselves from getting carried away by whatever attraction they feel. In Tantra there is no goal. The more we feel someone's beauty, their wholeness, the more we are drawn up into our own wholeness, a wholeness I am drawn up to again and again in front of masterpieces of art, a wholeness, the seeking of which, causes me to write some poems over and over, a practice that has carried over into developing forms and programs to realize the potential in Watsu and Tantsu.

ON THE SOURCES OF WATSU

The Ecstatic in the Creative- Light in Water...

Sitting in the house over a stream in which I sleep to the sound of running water, I look back on the sources of Watsu and see a child surrounded by water out on the tide flats of Whidbey Island, running up another flock of gulls, still following their flight up into that bright sky. I stoop over to scoop up another handful of sand to build another castle, knowing full well that, like all those before, it will soon disappear under the rising tide. Water takes so many shapes. Water has no shape.

I search my way through three college majors, Physics, Pre-Law, Philosophy, and finally find myself in the Creative Writing department at the University of Washington. I am a poet. And like most poets in 1957, on graduation, I head straight for San Francisco and, with great joy and great seriousness, dive headlong into the scene which us poets call the 'San Francisco Renaissance.'

In the poems that come to me, water or the sea and its waves are as common as being in love:

> How I am drawn back into that dark
> once more
> to stand on the shore
> before the mystery at the prow of Venus's bark
>
> as it scrapes sand and foamy dress thrown off
> she steps out.
> How I am drawn back to that spot
> I heard, running towards her new flowery dress, her cry and laugh
>
> Oh beauty born in the deep of night
> Oh beauty born of sexual delight.

I live on California's north coast, teach Pomo Indians in a one-room grade school and write. I cross another sea to Europe and immerse myself two years in its art and languages. I return to San Francisco… and the ocean at Stinson Beach:

> *Sanosa como la mar esta la nina*
> *Ay, Dios! Quien le hablaria?*

When she rode in on the wave and walked back smiling "It's beautiful. You really ride on top of the wave." I felt as good as if I had ridden in

and when after several failures trying as she said to 'get right there where the wave breaks' a wave carried me all the way in on top of it and I walked back to her she looked as happy as if she had ridden in

but when that 'right wave' I had waited so long for broke over me and the board broke under me against my balls and I jumped up in pain with only the top of the board in my hand in the froth beside me holding up the bottom she screamed

                "You broke it and I never got my turn again! You hogged it! You're so selfish! You would never let me have my turn and now you broke it!"

                and all the way up the shore all the way up to the men's showers she ran after me waving the bottom shouting riding on top of the crest of the wave of her anger

    Two years at Stinson Beach, three days a week I drive into San Francisco and study linguistics to complete my Masters in Teaching English as a Second Language. All year round, I go into the waves and bodysurf (without a board), without a wet suit, though Northern California waters are cold. But there is such ecstasy riding on these waves. I focus on the brightness in each wave and my body does not feel the cold. And one day, sitting out on a log over the ocean, the brightness of each wave's breaking becomes words breaking out of my mouth in languages I had never heard before, over and over, until all my questions are answered in one clear statement: 'Your voice is everybody's voice.'

    But that voice weakens- one year in Canada and three teaching at a University in Mexico City, the connection with that Ocean and the San Francisco Scene gradually dissolving. Without other poets to read and publish with, the poems come further and further apart. Returning to San Francisco, I feel even more isolated- North Beach emptied of its poets. I am not a flower child. I have always avoided psychedelics and psychotherapy and religion and whatever else might muddy the waters at the source of the poems, that clarity when the poem is writing itself with light. But that light is dim and those waters- more and more stagnant.

One day I discover that water comes in still another ecstatic form: hot springs. Out in the middle of the woods. How absolutely delicious to lie back in a pool of hot water naked under trees and sky, total peace. The next two years I scour the woods and mountains of California seeking out the wild ones. One day I ask a woman in one of the pools I find if she would like a massage. I am forty years old and have never received a massage in my life, let alone given one. She says yes and I start working on her back. She notices I'm not very experienced and shows me how to lift the shoulder blade to work under it. She knows massage. We become friends and, over the next few months, she teaches me. Having just built a hot spring like pool in my backyard, instead of buying a table, I set up a padded board just under its surface and massage people in warm water. I call it 'Wassage'.

My friend takes a course in Zen Shiatsu and sits me on the floor to give me a sample. I love it. I study with Reuho Yamada at his Temple of the Lotus Flowers, and Wataru Ohashi. I love the connection we feel when we lean into a point at the bottom of the breath. It is not unlike the peace at the center of the ecstasy in Tantra.

Hot springs create spontaneous community. They are wonderful places to find people to practice on. An offer to share Zen Shiatsu is always welcome. My favorite is Skagg's Springs. It is wild again after the last vestiges of a resort that had been condemned to make way for a reservoir have disappeared. One morning, sleeping beside the pool, I have a dream that wakes me to write:

> Snake shakes
> its diamonds in the water
>
> and all our loves
> shine and come out to play
>
> Snake shakes
> its diamonds in the water
>
> and all we have
> shimmers and flows away
>
> Snake shakes
> its diamonds in the water

Another morning before dawn I wake and go down to the pool. A woman is in it. I give her a Shiatsu while she sits in the water. When I finish she turns her head from side to side and says she hasn't been able to move like that since she had been in an accident. She says she felt healing in my hands. I thank her. My joy at hearing that stays with me as I stride up the side of a mountain, in awe that something like this could happen through me. At the top the circle of trees are filled with light. God is here. I drop to my knees. He bends down and lifts me. Holding my arm, He walks at my side along the ridge. He guides me down a stream. The streambed below is tangled in brush. There is an easier path along the gully's side. "Which way do I go?" "Whichever way you go I am with you." -words that never leave me. I sit out on the bank over the pool - such brightness- the pool, the children splashing in the water, the trees, the birds singing in the branches, are all sitting in God's hand. We are all sitting in God's hand. I look down at my own, open to hold others.

My beloved Skagg's is disappearing under the waters of a reservoir. Someone there once told me about another. Harbin Hot Springs is not wild (though some find it so), but it is a New Age workshop/retreat center with many people to practice Zen Shiatsu on. I complete my studies in Japan with my first two teachers' teacher, Shizuto Masunaga, and offer Zen Shiatsu workshops at Harbin. One night I float somebody in its warm pool and she floats me. My body starts to vibrate. I stand up and the vibrations are waves that rise up my back, all the way up into a world of light. I want to float others. I want to take others to that place. I float others and gradually incorporate stretches and moves from Zen Shiatsu, I call it Watsu.

ON THE SOURCES OF WATSU

Full Moon, July, 1983

If you happen to find your way into the warm pool at Harbin Hot Springs
and an old man with a white beard drifts up to your side
and, casually mentioning he comes up every weekend to teach the Shiatsu classes,
asks if you would like some in the water - 'Watsu' he calls it "something I developed
   in the pool here…I like to practice it every chance I get…"
accept
and you will find yourself being floated
your neck in the crook of his arm your sacrum in his hand
as he rocks you back and forth…back and around…back into a world without
   sound…back into the waters of the womb
as he swirls and sways you the way dolphins play
as he stretches leg and arm and back every way water allows
or drapes your legs over his shoulders and lifts you clear of it
the way an old man plays with the daughters of creation
and sets you down astraddle his held out leg
so that the chakra in your perineum is held from below by his thigh
and your hara by one hand
and your lower back by the other
so that the energy locked in that bowl is free to rise all the way up your spine
and join that old man's
two intertwining dragons spiraling heavenward…

Or
refuse.
Maybe he is just another lecherous old man
coming on
to all the pretty girls in the pool
"Thank you
I just want to be by myself…"
He
will find another
and another
and another
The sky is filled with dragons

That was fifteen years ago, in Watsu's Dragon Days, but in the days since, as Watsu spreads out into the wider world, most of those dragons are left up there with their tails hanging out of the sky. And rightly so. Each person's experience takes that form in which Spirit is ready to take, and it might not be a dragon. I've had to learn a lot about boundaries (which, had I learned earlier, would've stopped me from floating anybody. In the nineties I'm not comfortable going up to a stranger.) One of the first lessons I learned was that what I perceive as waves of energy rising up into light, is not necessarily perceived that way by others. I used to end each session holding my partner to share those waves rising up. Then one day I held someone who has had a history of abuse. I quickly changed that ending to today's, where we leave a person in their own space against the wall and focus on the connection we still have without any physical contact. This is right. I had made that rising of light at the end a goal. Watsu has no goal.

There was little stillness in the Dragon Watsus. There was no Water Breath Dance…no listening… no Follow Movement. These came later- the stillness that the other can drop deepest into and find where their own wave and rising begins. And if they do, it is then, resonating to that, being with the other, that our own wave can reach its highest. And if they don't, we stay in the stillness with them. This is right. Watsus are still poems written in water, but they are poems we write together.

A footnote on the Body Wave

Those who see it or feel it in another without having experienced it in their own body, may interpret it as sexual or worse. In the Middle Ages, women who had these kinds of waves were burned as witches. In the 19th century Anton Mesmer had to cut short his pioneering work with energy in Paris because the medical establishment, seeing a woman he touched go into waves, made a law against it saying it was unhealthy for both the patient and the practitioner. Recently in India, a Yoga teacher, known around the world for the control over the body he exhibits and demands, after repeatedly telling a student to stop her belly's vibrating when she went into a pose, stepped up and kicked it.

The wave is a letting go of control; the wave that connects us to those we hold close to our heart, the wave that rises up out of the void we drop deepest into in meditation. Wherever control is let go of in the continuing creation that is this universe, a new order spontaneously arises. That wave or spiral up into light is that most basic principal of creation being actualized within us again and again- light in water. This is where Watsu began for me.

A footnote to the footnote

where Watsu began for me… and where does it stop? Where do the ripples sent out from that first pebble stop. Ripples? Hardly had that pebble hit the water and someone picked up someone in their arms and jumped in, and those in their arms picked up someone and jumped in- and at this moment, and at every moment, someone, somewhere around the world, is picking up someone in their arms and jumping in. So much light in the water. It never goes out. A wave that never breaks. A World Wave that we are all in the arms of- the whole Water Family.

WORLDWIDE AQUATIC BODYWORK REGISTRY

More than 30 years ago when I began teaching Watsu and Tantsu around the world I started a Registry that stored the transcripts of our students and made it possible for them to study with different instructors in different countries and apply those studies to authorizations on the Registry as practitioners and instructors.

Today 20,000 students from more than 95 countries have transcripts on the Registry. More than a hundred Instructors of Watsu, other aquatic modalities, and Tantsu post their classes and students on the Registry. When you take a class, it is added to your transcript. Each authorization to practice or teach is added. Once you are authorized, as long as you maintain our ethical standards, meet continuing education requirements, and remain a member of WABA you may choose to be listed to the public on the Registry and have your transcripts visible to those seeking practitioners and instructors on the internet.

The Registry provides feedback about each instructor's courses. It works closely with training institutes in several countries that post their classes and students.

It maintains a message board for those on the Registry and a list of available pools. WABA, a not for profit member association, that includes all current practitioners and instructors works closely with the Registry.

Watsu and Tantsu are trademarked. Whenever you consider taking an Aquatic Bodywork class, check to see if is listed on the Registry. If not, its instructor may not be fully trained and authorized and the class can not be added to your transcript and applied to future classes or authorizations

www.watsu.com

Books

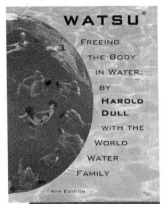

This book is out of print.
It is being replaced by a companion volume to this book:

Watsu Professional Path

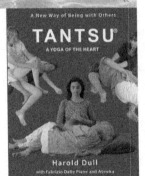

THE TANTSU PATHS This English edition appeared concurrently with the edition commissioned in Italy where its 300 colored illustrations were photographed. Step by step it presents the holds and moves of the new Core Tantsu that can be shared with friends, a Tantsu for Partners, and the Traditional Tantsu used in a professional practice. Fabrizio Dalle Piane and Ateeka, who helped Harold develop the new Core Tantsu, have contributed insightful articles that investigate Tantsu's place among other disciplines that explore our movement within. 112 pages.

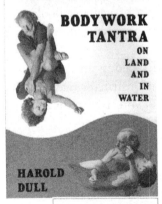

FIRST FIRST WATSU TANTSU PATHS Copies of Harold's first Watsu and Tantsu book, ***Bodywork Tantra***,1987. Collector's items.

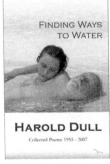

FINDING WAYS TO WATER This book combines all of Harold's poetry from his days as a poet in the San Francisco Renaissance to those inspired by Watsu (which is itself poetry in water). Collected Poems 1955-2007 ... 208 pages. His reading of it is available on a CD. Some are available at www.watsu.com/harold.

DVDs

Watsu 1 *2012*
- New Basic
- New Transition Flow.
- Tantsuyoga..
- Flower Round.

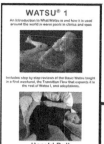

Watsu 2
- Expanded Flow: bodywork and stretches to expand the Transition Flow.
- Adaptations.
- Underwater footage.

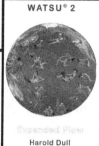

Watsu 3
- Powerful stretches and other Advanced Moves including those done on the steps.
- Rolls that introduce Free Flow (from dozens of actual sessions).

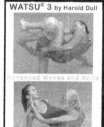

Tantsu and Home Spa Watsu
- A complete traditional Tantsu.
- Watsu in a Jacuzzi.
- Tantsu by two.
- Combine Zen Shiatsu and Tantsu.

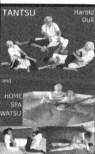

Core Tantsu
- How its whole body cradles' containment frees our inner dance.
- A step by step progression of simple and comfortable moves.

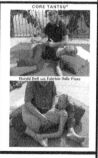

Tantsuyoga and Tandem Watsu
- Tantsuyoga Flower Rounds.
- Tantsuyoga by Two
- Tandem Watsu.

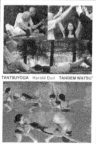

Downloadable videos will be available.

Order Books and DVDs from Watsu Publishing www.watsu.com (707) 684 0207

ONE WATER FAMILY WORLDWIDE

Worldwide Aquatic Bodywork Association

The non-profit Worldwide Aquatic Bodywork Association oversees aquatic bodywork training and certification programs and their ethical application; coordinates research; and helps provide access to the benefits of aquatic bodywork. Practitioners, Instructors, and Training Institutes listed on the Worldwide Registry are members of WABA. Other individuals and organizations who want to help are welcome to become WABA members.

Afterwords

For me, this new version, starts to complete my part in realizing the potential of what was put into my hands (or rather into my arms) almost 40 years ago. With the Water Family's help Watsu's role in helping clients through a growing number of conditions in clinics and spas around the world has been established. This book presents something that can help free us from the one condition we all suffer, separation, or rather the illusion of separation. The first books focus on what Watsu and Tantsu can do for others, this book on their potential to bring everyone, everywhere, closer together to discover again what we don't know we know.

More than 60 years ago I started writing the poetry that took my life onto a new course, a course that seemed moved away from when I started taking people into the water, but now writing my way a seventh time through this book, I see that the wholeness that has always meant the most to me in poems and works of art and the universe is what we hold when we hold others on this path. It is one path.

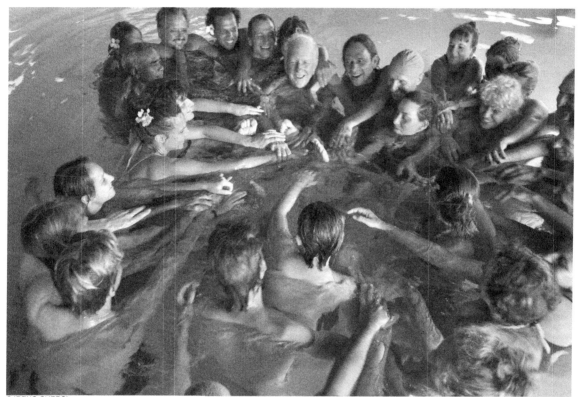
© IRENO GUERCI

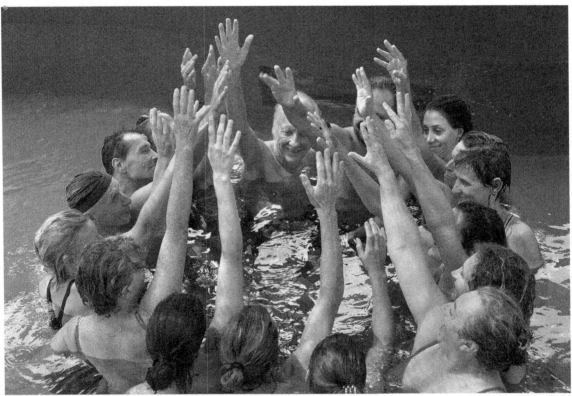
© IRENO GUERCI

Made in the USA
Middletown, DE
21 May 2023

31122928R00097